THE RUNNER'S COMPLETE MEDICAL GUIDE

RICHARD MANGI, M.D.
PETER JOKL, M.D.
O. WILLIAM DAYTON

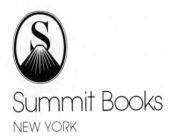

Summit Books
NEW YORK

Acknowledgment:

The authors are grateful to Dave Dushkin for his assistance with the manuscript, and to Virginia Simon and Heidi Humphrey for their help with the illustrations.

Copyright © 1979 by Richard Mangi, M.D., Peter Jokl, M.D., and O. William Dayton

Published by *Summit Books*
A Simon & Schuster Division of Gulf & Western Corporation
Simon & Schuster Building
1230 Avenue of the Americas
New York, New York 10020
SUMMIT BOOKS and colophon are trademarks
of Simon & Schuster
Designed by Stanley S. Drate
Manufactured in the United States of America
    2 3 4 5 6 7 8 9 10
2 3 4 5 6 7 8 9 10 11 Pbk.

Library of Congress Cataloging in Publication Data

Mangi, Richard.
    The runner's complete medical guide.

    Bibliography: p.
    Includes index.
    1. Running—Physiological aspects. 2. Running
—Accidents and injuries—Prevention. 3. Sports
medicine. I. Jokl, Peter, joint author.
II. Dayton, O. William, joint author.
III. Title.
RC1220.R8M36   617'.1027   79-15874

ISBN 0-671-40096-7
ISBN 0-671-40118-1 Pbk.

Contents

1

Let the Runner Beware

Runners are the fittest group of sick and injured people in the world. While running is probably the most natural and healthful sport ever played, its participants must frequently push their mental and physical capacities to the limit. Every year a few hapless runners are hospitalized with serious complications from their sport. Recently three Japanese runners actually died from heatstroke during a hot weather marathon. Every runner on the face of the earth has experienced less severe problems such as blisters, muscle pulls, tendinitis, stress fractures, sprains or dog bites. To achieve the full benefits from running, be they recreational or competitive, runners must understand their bodies and keenly watch for subtle signs of injury and disease. Running should be a lifelong pursuit. No race or training schedule is so important that a runner should gamble his future health.

Despite efforts to stereotype runners, they are a very mixed group. No two have the same running style or body build, and each one will have individual medical problems and running injuries. Some require the professional help of a podiatrist, others an orthopedic surgeon, and still others a cardiologist or an athletic trainer. No one professional group can solve all the potential problems that an individual runner may develop. With this realization, we saw the need for a book that would provide runners with basic scientific and medical information to be used for prevention and early treatment of medical problems and injuries. Our aim is to help runners recognize and deal with a wide spectrum of medical problems. Richard Mangi is a specialist in internal medicine: the basic functions and diseases of the human body. Peter Jokl is an orthopedic surgeon and specialist in athletic injuries. Bill Dayton is an athletic trainer: a specialist in the prevention, early treatment and rehabilitation of athletic injuries. Mangi and Jokl are avid long distance runners, and Dayton has been treating injured runners for over forty years. While our training and experience is quite different, we share a basic concern and interest in running as a sport, a profession, and a way of life. We therefore understand the needs of runners, as well as the concerns of their doctors. Our philosophy is to keep a runner running whenever possible. We encourage sick or injured runners to resume running as soon as possible. But we realize the consequences of an improperly treated injury, and we refuse to sacrifice a runner's health and future career for the sake of a single race.

Sports medicine is still in its infancy. Honest controversy abounds, and this debate is healthy for the future. We have attempted to keep an open mind and to approach problems in a logical and scientific manner. Since we have no ax to grind, we have tried to give the reader a balanced picture of controversial topics, but we cannot condone a fringe element philosophy embraced by those who promote their own beliefs at the expense of accepted medical wisdom.

An intelligent runner should be able to separate quackery, gimmickry and fraud from honest professional opinion. Skepticism is a healthy virtue. Don't believe anything until you examine solid evidence. Even everyday accepted medical care is burdened by rituals and habits that have no basis in fact. A quick glance at a few "scientific facts" of the past will confirm this theory. Today we laugh at leeching, the vapors, bad night air and the like. George Washington developed a strep throat and was bled to death by the most eminent physicians of his day. We can assume that people of the twenty-first century will find as much humor in our "modern medicine." Quacks, observing the flaws of modern medicine, claim that doctors are fools, and that only they know the real answer. Rational runners, however, understand that medicine is an inexact science. At the same time, they realize that doctors are professionals, trained in the scientific methods, with a healthy respect for education and an open mind to new facts.

We don't claim to know the value of brewer's yeast, megavitamins, juice fasts, bee pollens or high protein diets. But the promoters of these fads do. They make a lot of money from gullible runners. If you wish to waste money on fads, please be honest with yourself. Remember the main advantage is purely psychological, and that's what you're paying for. Common sense is particularly valuable in this instance, for some fads, such as liquid protein diets, are dangerous and possibly fatal. With a little practice it's easy to spot a charlatan. Beware of:

- Anyone who claims to have the only answer
- Quick "magic" cures
- Anyone who ridicules honest professionals and praises himself
- Aids, pills, and supplements promoted by slick advertisements
- Anything that offends your common sense

Instead, learn how a runner's body functions, how it adapts to training, and how it develops disease. A runner is born with the basic equipment of his sport. He can't use fiberglass legs and a graphite heart. He must use his own body; nothing else matters very much. This stark simplicity is one of the most appealing elements of running. But the human body is a complex machine, and a smart runner uses his knowledge of its workings to his own advantage.

Too frequently, runners and doctors develop an adversary relationship. A doctor may not understand a runner's need to run despite an injury or an illness, while some runners develop "superman complexes" and think themselves immune to disease. Being both a doctor and a runner, I can say that neither group is always right. My point is not that doctors don't know what they're doing. To the contrary, they almost always work with the highest level of skill and integrity. But they are human.

They don't know what they haven't been taught or haven't learned by experience. Running is still a new sport in this country. As it grows in popularity, medical knowledge and experience in the treatment of runners' diseases will also grow. Runners should help foster this process. They should learn about other runners' problems and diseases and share their own experiences so that others might benefit. In the meantime, there are several things an individual runner can do to guarantee the best care for himself.

Always seek help from experienced professionals—medical doctors, surgeons, podiatrists or athletic trainers. If you're lucky, someone in your city knows how to treat runners' ailments. Ask other runners. They are universally helpful and usually know who can best help you.

Don't be fooled by fancy titles and certificates. Anyone can call himself a specialist in sports medicine or runners' diseases. Discover for yourself if this person really knows the sport and understands your interests and needs. Politely inquire about his experience treating other runners and athletes. An honest person will gladly supply this information.

Avoid anyone who claims that only he can help you. Nobody knows everything, particularly about a field as complicated as the human body. Beware of statements like "All runners' problems begin and end with the foot," or "Only an orthopedic surgeon can treat an athlete."

If you can't find a professional who is experienced in runners' ailments, stick with your family doctor. If you trust him and he is willing to try, then you can help each other to learn. Read books, ask other runners, call up people in other cities. One great trait of runners is their eagerness to help each other. If you're persistent, you'll find somebody who knows how to help you. Bring this information to your doctor. He'll be grateful and so will his other patients who run.

The Runner's Complete Medical Guide is divided into two parts: Runners' Injuries and Runners' Medical Problems. Chapters are organized in a system-oriented approach. Each chapter covers a separate body organ or region of anatomy. To orient the reader, we begin with a brief outline of the structure and function of a particular organ, followed by changes that occur during running and adaptations to training. A list of diseases or injuries then follows. The cause, symptoms and diagnostic methods for each ailment are listed, followed by treatment recommendations and other pertinent comments for runners. Other diseases worthy of brief mention are listed at the end of each chapter.

The book is designed as a reference for runners, trainers, coaches, and medical professionals of all types. It should be used as an aid in diagnosing, treating and preventing specific runners' medical problems and injuries. We do not intend it to be a comprehensive medical text. The emphasis is placed on injuries and diseases caused or aggravated by running. But many common diseases are also included because runners who suffer from these ailments often ask how this condition affects running and vice versa.

We have tried to present the information in this book factually. Theories and fads are described as such, letting the reader draw his own conclusions. Much of medical care is still an inexact science, or art, if you will. There are many ways to treat a blister or to recover from an injury. We present the methods which we prefer, based on our personal experience. If you or your doctor use another approach, fine—as long as you get the results you want. Moreover, if you are not helped by our recommendations, please seek the opinion of other professionals. Nothing works all the time for everybody.

Running and running medicine are our lifelong avocations. We would appreciate hearing from other runners and professionals regarding their ailments and experiences so that we may all profit in the end.

2

Avoiding Injuries

The average runner sustains at least one serious injury a year. Injuries are certainly not a sign of mediocrity. In fact many of the world's best runners are just as frequently sidelined by these problems. Not only do injuries interrupt training schedules, but they may also be psychologically devastating. It takes about three days of training to make up one day lost to injury. More important, an injury that ruins a runner's chance for a state championship or an Olympic medal can permanently destroy his mental attitude. It is not unusual for a first-class runner never to "recover" from a seemingly minor injury, and many great athletic careers have ended prematurely.

Obviously no one likes to be injured, yet a surprising number of runners at all levels simply ignore ways to prevent injuries. Most can be avoided completely or at least controlled by adhering to certain basic principles and using a sensible approach to training. Injuries often occur when a runner neglects any one of the following:

- Adequate conditioning
- Sufficient warm-up and cool-down periods
- Proper running style
- Adequate equipment

- Attention to mechanical and environmental problems
- Treatment of minor injuries

CONDITIONING

Physical conditioning is the end result of long months of train-ing. Arthur Lydiard's adage to "train, don't strain" is a concise summary of the basic philosophy of all conditioning programs. A runner's body changes in many ways during training. Each organ of the body must adapt slowly to the stresses demanded by running. After a training session, there must be a rest period to allow the body to recover, adapt and become stronger. As the work load is slowly increased during subsequent training ses-sions, the body will be able to tolerate greater and greater stresses. Never exceed the capacity of the body during a training program. When too large a stress is placed on the body, an "over-use" injury will occur.

There are a wide variety of training programs, but all share three basic goals: increased strength, endurance and speed.

Strength

Muscle strength increases the power of a runner's stride and lengthens his gait. While it is more important for sprinters than for long distance runners, all runners will benefit from stronger leg muscles. Strength can be developed by weight training, re-sistance workouts such as running up hills, and to some extent by long distance running. The great majority of distance runners gain adequate strength for competition by long distance training alone. Weight training, however, is a much quicker method and has been used to advantage by many world class runners. Coaches debate its value for the average runner, but most agree that sprinters and some distance runners improve from weight training, especially to increase upper body strength.

If a runner plans a weight program, the exercises should be performed slowly and deliberately and should include approxi-mately three sets of ten repetitions of each exercise. Weight ex-ercises should not be done more frequently than every other day. One of the pitfalls of weight conditioning is strengthening one muscle group without strengthening the opposite muscles. Muscle imbalance results, leading to injuries. For example, sprinters may overdevelop quadriceps muscles without strengthening their hamstrings, thereby increasing their chance of hamstring injuries (see Chapter 9).

Most coaches prefer to strengthen leg muscles by resistance running. Running up hills or on soft surfaces, such as sand, are the two most commonly used methods of resistance running. Both will rapidly increase muscle strength and endurance.

Endurance

Endurance is the ability of muscles to perform repetitive work over a long period of time. It is a specific biochemical process with muscle enzyme changes (described in Chapter 4). All runners must develop endurance to a certain extent by one of the basic methods: long distance running, high repetition interval running, weight training or resistance running.

Most prefer long distance running as the foundation of endurance. Therefore, endurance is closely tied to the aerobic base: the number of miles run per week at a comfortable pace, during which the exercise does not use up more oxygen than the lungs can supply. A good aerobic base strengthens the muscles, joints, tendons, ligaments and cardiovascular system, all of which are essential for endurance. There is no shortcut to building this base. Generally, weekly mileage should be increased by no more than 10–15 percent a month. Most coaches also recommend that long distance runners include a 20-mile run each week to insure maximum endurance, and scientific studies confirm this advice. Runs of this distance deplete muscle glycogen and stimulate fatty acid metabolism (see Chapter 4), changes that are essential for maximum endurance.

Devotees of interval training claim that high levels of endurance can be gained by massive doses of interval running. Their schedules may consist of repetitive speed runs of 220, 440, or 880 yards or more. Undoubtedly, this method has proved successful. The famous Emil Zatopek is the most illustrious example of the endurance benefits of massive interval work. Since runners often find it difficult to run 15–20 miles of intervals on a track, most coaches discourage this type of endurance training.

While weight training and resistance running are strengthening exercises, they will develop muscle endurance only to a limited extent. These workouts must be combined with long distance running, intervals or some other form of endurance training.

Speed

Speed is the ability to run faster over a given distance. It can be considered in terms of neuromuscular coordination, anaerobic fitness and pace.

Neuromuscular coordination is the basic property necessary for speed. The legs must be moved quickly and efficiently. Much of this ability is inborn, but it is one talent that can be improved by training. Hours of repetitive running at any speed will teach the body how to move more efficiently, and with time, runners are able to move over the ground with less work. To go beyond efficiency and actually increase leg and ankle speed, however, a runner must periodically set a faster-than-race pace. This workout can be done on the track in the form of short distance intervals or sprints, or during longer runs as pace work, speeding up from time to time.

Anaerobic fitness defines the ability to run while the body uses more oxygen than the lungs are able to take in. Obviously, anaerobic running can be continued only for a relatively short period of time. A runner, however, can condition himself to tolerate this "oxygen debt" for longer and longer periods of time. Fast pace interval running is the basic method of anaerobic training. After each interval, the body is allowed to recover the oxygen debt by resting or running slowly for a short distance. After several weeks of anaerobic training, a runner is able to perform for a longer distance under anaerobic conditions.

Pace is a crucial element of speed in races of almost any distance. Clearly, any mediocre runner can run 110 yards in 15 seconds. But it takes a better runner to run a quarter mile in 60 seconds and an elite runner to run a 4-minute mile. Ideally, a runner will pace himself by proportioning his energy equally throughout a race, so that he reaches the exact limit of his capacity at the moment he hits the finish line. Proper pacing can be considered the most important element of speed, particularly in long distance races. Runners usually develop pace by running at race pace over shorter than race distances. For example, a miler planning to run a 4-minute mile may run repetitive 60-second quarters, while a marathoner shooting for a 2:10 marathon may run 10–20 kilometers at a 5-minute-per-mile pace. The pace plans of many beginning runners are destroyed by the excitement at the start of a race. They run the first half of a race too fast and are then too exhausted to maintain that pace to the finish line. Racing is actually one of the best ways of learning to pace yourself. Low-key races at distances less than your intended specialty are particularly helpful and enjoyable too.

An intelligent runner will decide exactly what he is trying to accomplish as a runner. He will gear his overall training and each workout accordingly. Proper training programs should include the right balance of strengthening, endurance training and speed work. A sprinter concentrates on strength, speed and anaerobic fitness, while a marathon runner is more concerned with endurance and pacing. In addition to these general considerations, most runners should divide the year into different training seasons. They should plan a basic aerobic conditioning period, during which the body is allowed to develop strength and endurance by slow-to-moderate-pace long distance running. A 2–3 month precompetitive season should follow, during which the body is trained for speed, endurance and pace. At the end of the preseason, a 6–8 week sharpening period should bring physical conditioning to a peak, as anaerobic fitness, leg speed and pace training are emphasized. The principle of gradually applied stress is particularly important at this time. If minor injuries, muscle soreness, fatigue or other signs of staleness develop, the work load should be temporarily decreased. During the competitive season, runners strive to maintain peak form for important races. There is a fine line between peak conditioning and injury. Races place excessive stress on the body and very few runners can compete at 100 percent effort for long without developing injuries. Beginning runners should carefully plan a modest racing season at first, going all out in only one or two important races. Once an individual's limitations are clearly defined, his competitive season can be lengthened. The post-competitive season should be a rest period relegated to relaxed fun-running with no specific training goals. This type of running helps condition the body with a minimum risk of injury.

WARM-UP AND COOL-DOWN

The value of warm-up has been clearly established by scientific studies. Runners who warm up before every workout and race have a definite competitive advantage. During exercise, muscles generate heat from metabolic processes. After 15–20 minutes of warm-up exercises, muscle temperatures rise a few degrees and muscles will perform more efficiently. In addition, during the warm-up period, blood vessels shunt blood to exercising muscle groups; the heart and lungs adjust to the increased demands of running; and muscles, tendons and ligaments are gently stretched, minimizing the risk of injury during a race. A warm-up period should be individualized to meet the specific requirements of the runner. Stretching exercises, however, are an essential element of the warm-up and cool-down as well as of proper conditioning. Basic stretching routines are outlined in Figure 2-1. A runner should stretch each major running muscle group daily. Warm-up exercises should be performed prior to every workout and should include at least 5 minutes of gradual stretching followed by a brief but brisk walk or slow jog. Pace should be increased gradually for the first 15 minutes. As a good rule of thumb, a runner should exercise for at least 15 minutes prior to a speed workout or a race, and should be sweating gently, his heart and breathing rate already increased at the start of a workout or starting line of a race.

A cool-down period is also an integral part of proper running. After a workout or race, a runner should walk or slowly jog for a few minutes, followed by a routine of stretching exercises. This practice helps to prevent tight muscles and promotes removal of waste products. Runners who cool down note less muscle soreness the day after a hard workout.

RUNNING STYLE

There is a tremendous variation in running style among runners of all abilities. Although there are many ways to get the job

stretching exercises

Stretching exercises should be performed slowly with few repetitions several times a day. Remember, you can overstretch!

hamstrings

exercise one

1. Spread legs 24" apart.
2. Bend over (knees stiff).
3. S t r e t c h (do not bounce).
4. Return to upright position.

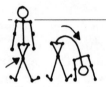

exercise two

1. Cross feet.
2. Bend over to touch floor.
3. s t r e t c h
4. Return to upright position.
5. Change feet and repeat.

exercise three

1. Standing on one leg, place opposite heel on table about 30" high.
2. Bend at waist and touch toes (keep knees stiff).
3. s t r e t c h
4. Return to upright position.
5. Change legs.

exercise four

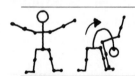

1. Spread feet 24" apart.
2. Bring arms out at shoulder level.
3. Twist and bend, touching fingers to opposite foot.
4. Return to upright position.
5. Alternate.

exercise five

1. Sit on floor with one leg extended, one flexed at side.
2. Grasp toes.
3. Pull body toward toes.
4. Alternate.

exercise six

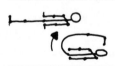

1. Lie flat on back, with hands at side.
2. Roll legs up and over head.
3. Touch floor above head.
4. Return legs to lying position.
5. Repeat.

Figure 2-1

quadriceps

exercise one

1. Lie on front.
2. Reach back and hold ankle.
3. Pull heel to buttocks. Do not jerk!
4. Return to floor.
5. Alternate.

exercise two

1. Sit on floor, with one leg extended, one flexed at side.
2. Lie back on floor.
3. Return to upright position.
4. Alternate.

exercise three

1. A rather tough exercise for the quads. It also stretches ligaments around the ankles. Not too highly recommended.

exercise four

1. The same as quad exercise one but standing. Many people use this as a quad stretcher, but in this exercise the pelvis moves and you do not get the full stretch. We suggest exercise one instead.

heel cord

exercise one

1. Stand about 30" from wall.
2. Lean to wall at arm's length.
3. Push abdomen towards wall, keeping knees stiff.
4. Return and repeat.

exercise two

1. Same as exercise one, except swivel pelvis from side to side.
2. Repeat.

exercise three

1. Same as exercise one, except flex one knee.
2. Repeat.

Figure 2-1 (continued).

achilles tendon

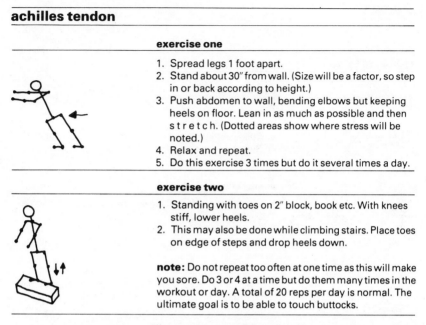

exercise one

1. Spread legs 1 foot apart.
2. Stand about 30" from wall. (Size will be a factor, so step in or back according to height.)
3. Push abdomen to wall, bending elbows but keeping heels on floor. Lean in as much as possible and then s t r e t c h. (Dotted areas show where stress will be noted.)
4. Relax and repeat.
5. Do this exercise 3 times but do it several times a day.

exercise two

1. Standing with toes on 2" block, book etc. With knees stiff, lower heels.
2. This may also be done while climbing stairs. Place toes on edge of steps and drop heels down.

note: Do not repeat too often at one time as this will make you sore. Do 3 or 4 at a time but do them many times in the workout or day. A total of 20 reps per day is normal. The ultimate goal is to be able to touch buttocks.

Figure 2-1 (continued).

done, this does not necessarily mean that anything goes. Many injuries are due to improper running technique, and recurrent injuries can often be cured by evaluating and correcting running style. One should generally not copy the style of another runner because what may be natural and economical for one person may not be right for another.

There are, however, certain accepted basic principles. The body should be upright with the pelvis tipped forward. The feet should strike the ground directly below the body. Overstriding is uneconomical and can damage the shins and knees. Stride length should be approximately equal to a runner's height. More experienced runners favor shorter strides which are apparently more economical. Foot plant is extremely important. Most authorities agree that the toes should point straight ahead, and the feet should land so that the footprints line up exactly. This "tightrope running" is a mark of all good distance runners. On a dirt track or sandy beach, a straight line drawn from the start to the finish should intersect the center of each footprint. When a runner points his toes outward in a ducklike gait, the stride will be naturally shortened. In addition, these runners have a very high incidence of shin splints. Not surprisingly, there is still considerable debate as to the ideal foot plant. While authorities also agree that sprinters and most middle distance runners land on the ball of the foot, there is still not uniform agreement as to the best method for distance runners. Most joggers and fun-runners should land on the outside of the heel, rolling their weight along the side of the foot onto the ball or metatarsals. This heel-toe strike causes less injuries than metatarsal or flat-foot-type foot plants. The toe-runner who lands on the ball of the foot and gradually shifts his weight back to the heel frequently develops tightness and soreness of the calf muscles. The flatfoot or clog-type gait causes excessive jarring of the ankles, knees and hips.

Many beginning runners suffer from another stylistic problem. They run with straight legs, not raising their knees high enough to get their feet far from the ground. As a result their hips rotate and their legs and feet swivel off to the side like windmills. This clumsy gait produces zig-zag running as well as an increased risk of injuries to the knees and hips.

Hold the arms in the most comfortable position. While there is considerable variation, the forearms should generally be parallel with the ground and the hands should swing in an arc from the side seam of the pants directly forward 12–18 inches. Arm motion helps body balance and hip excursion, and is therefore desirable, but should come from a flexible elbow with relatively little movement of the shoulders. Tight, high arm carriage, locked elbows, dipping shoulders and forearms that flail out to the side or in across the body are common beginner faults, which waste energy and cause premature tiring. The wrists should be firm so that the hands do not flop, but the fingers should be loose and relaxed. Usually arms are carried lower while running uphill and higher when running downhill.

One of the most important elements of good running style is the ability to relax while running. Many unhappy beginners complain of "tying up" during a race. The body's muscles tense during competition, restricting normal motion and thereby inhibiting running speed. Relaxation is also important to prevent injuries because tense muscles and joints are more prone to injury. It comes with experience and practice, and beginners should consciously try to relax each muscle of their bodies until it becomes part of their running form.

EQUIPMENT

Good equipment is essential for prevention of injuries in every sport. Runners perform with a minimum of equipment which is part of the sport's great appeal. A good pair of running shoes is the basic requirement. There are at least a dozen good training and racing shoes on the market. Decide on your own particular needs and then pick the shoe that best fits these requirements. Do not make the mistake of buying shoes solely on the basis of style or national ratings. The first basic principle is fit. Some companies make shoes in narrow widths only, and runners with wide feet must avoid these brands regardless of how well an Olympic medalist performs in them. The reverse is just as important. People with narrow feet, particularly women, should not buy wide shoes. Shoes that are too big are just as dangerous as shoes that are too small. Heavier runners and runners who spend most of their time running on cement and other hard surfaces should purchase shoes with ample cushioning.

A shoe should be snug and comfortable (Figure 2-2). Both shoes of a pair should be tried on, for feet are not always the same size. The most important factor determining the choice of training shoes should be protection from injuries. Most training shoes are heavy because of the added support features. The sole should be flexible and somewhat spongy. While there are two types of sponge—one very soft and the other firmer in consistency—the firmer sponge sole is generally preferable in a training shoe because of the added protection to the metatarsals. This is particularly important for individuals who run over trails or irregular terrain where there is danger of stepping on rocks and other irregular objects. The sponge sole should extend all the way from heel to toe. The front part of the shoe should be flexible. A stiff shank is most important for the heel-to-toe type of running that is the basis of training. Most shoes contain a built-in arch support which can be removed if you are more comfortable without it. The heel should be snug. If it is too wide, the foot will wiggle, causing calluses or blisters.

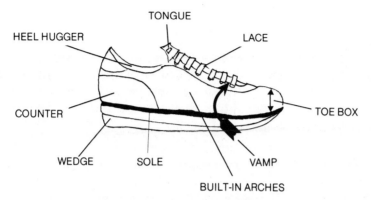

Running Shoe Components

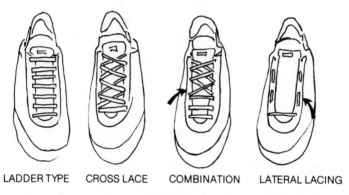

Shoe Lacing

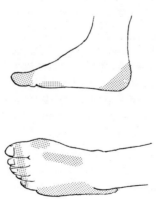

Most common sites of friction from running shoes

Figure 2-2.   RUNNING SHOES

Many runners rotate training shoes and sometimes use more than one brand. Rotation of brands is occasionally desirable because the slightly different contours, arch supports and soles of different brands cause slightly different stresses on the feet and calves. For example, a runner who trains solely in a shoe with a high heel can develop tightness of the calf muscles. Running in a shoe with a low arch and heel will stretch the calf. Rotation allows shoes to dry out completely between workouts and also helps prevent blisters from minor pressure points that vary from shoe to shoe.

Socks should fit snugly without wrinkling. The tube sock is excellent in this regard. If socks are too tight, they can cause ingrown toenails and blisters. Many runners wear two pairs of socks, a light nylon pair inside the heavier cotton athletic sock. Others prefer to run with no socks at all, lubricating their toes with lanolin or petroleum jelly to minimize friction and prevent blisters.

Style of shirts and shorts are an individual preference. They should fit properly and not cause irritation or friction.

MECHANICAL AND ENVIRONMENTAL PROBLEMS

In addition to the specific problems discussed later, runners should adopt certain general safety principles. Always carry identification in case of an accident. "Medic-Alert"-type bracelets should be worn by persons with diabetes, drug allergies or other special problems. When a runner plans a run, especially alone, he should always tell family or friends what his expected route is and when he plans to return. Always plan to stop somewhere for water, particularly during hot weather. It is also useful to carry some money in case of an emergency. It is not wise to take solitary runs into the wilderness. If an accident occurs, it's a great relief to have a companion to send for help.

Running Surfaces

Many injuries are related to the type of surface used in training. Hard ones like cement jar the legs, causing muscle soreness and foot, tendon and joint injuries. Asphalt is softer than cement. Running on roads, however, causes knee and ankle injuries because of the shape of the pavement. Most roads are turtle-backed, sloping to either side. Unless a runner stays in the middle of the road, one foot lands lower than the other. This uneven running places excessive stress on the uphill leg and outward rotation of the downhill leg (see Figure 2-3). It is therefore wise to try to run in the middle of the road when there is no traffic. During the summer when the asphalt is hot, road runners frequently develop blisters of the feet.

Soft surfaces such as grass and dirt generally cause less shock to the body and, therefore, less injuries. These surfaces have resilience and keep spring in the legs. A runner should try to train at least a few days a week on a soft surface. Parks, golf courses, infields of tracks and dirt roads are all good places for this type of training. Running over undulating terrain such as a golf course is a particularly good conditioning practice, for runners must vary their strides, thereby exercising many different muscle groups. However, these surfaces can be hazardous since a careless runner can sprain or break his ankle by stepping into a hole or twisting his foot on a loose rock.

Running in sand is excellent for building strength and endurance, but it frequently causes muscle tightness and shortening. Sand workouts should always be followed by proper stretching.

Running on tracks, particularly small indoor tracks, often causes injuries. The narrow turns interrupt the normal fluid motion of running. A runner tends to lean into a turn causing extra stress on his inside leg. Soreness of the foot and ankle frequently occurs. Whenever possible, change direction from time to time. Runners often warm up in one direction and perform interval work in the opposite one.

Weather Conditions

Running in the rain is enjoyable, but a runner should be sure that his shoes have adequate soles to prevent him from slipping. Waffle- or stud-type soles are usually best. Avoid puddles for fear of a hidden pothole. An icy surface is particularly dangerous

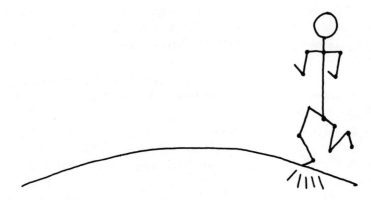

Right Leg. May be injured from excessive stress on uphill extremity. Calf, knee or hip damage may result from jarring of right side.

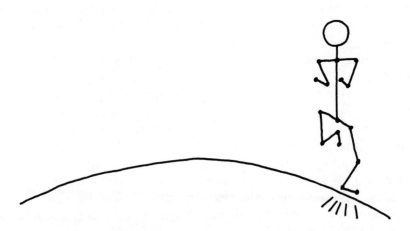

Left Leg. May be injured by external rotation of hip and improper foot plant. Shin splints may also result from improper foot plant. Uneven strain on abductor muscles may cause pain on outside of knee.

Figure 2-3.   ROAD RUNNING AGAINST TRAFFIC

and should be avoided at all costs. Remember that rain or snow limits visibility and wear brightly colored clothing under these conditions to make yourself plainly visible to automobile drivers.

Lightning kills many persons each year. Outdoor athletes, like runners, are frequently exposed to lightning or thunderstorms. Never begin a run in this kind of storm. If caught outside, seek shelter in a sturdy building if you can. Avoid open fields and trees. Lightning causes stoppage of the heart, which can often be reversed through immediate attention. If a running companion is hit by lightning, immediately begin cardiopulmonary resuscitation until medical help arrives. Most communities offer courses teaching the life-saving techniques of mouth-to-mouth resuscitation and external cardiac massage.

Heat is probably the most dangerous weather condition confronting runners. Humidity compounds this problem. (Hot weather diseases are discussed in detail in Chapter 18.)

Cold weather can tighten muscles and tendons leading to injuries. Be particularly careful to warm up slowly and completely especially before racing in cold temperatures. Frostbite of the penis (Chapter 17) and dead fingers (Chapter 12) are also complications of cold weather running. To keep warm during cold weather, use several layers of thin clothing. Nylon garments are particularly useful because they preserve body heat and are an excellent barrier to wind. Runners' asthma is a medical disease frequently aggravated by cold weather (Chapter 14).

Running at a high altitude is an excellent way to train before a major race. The low oxygen content of high altitude air stimulates the body to produce more red blood cells. These extra blood cells carry more oxygen to the body, increasing running ability. Runners should allow their bodies to adjust slowly to altitude training. However, it takes 2–3 weeks to acclimate to high altitudes. Decrease the usual training schedule at first and avoid hard workouts for at least 2 weeks. Altitude sickeness is a common problem encountered by individuals who travel to high elevations. Headache, nausea and dizziness develop and are aggravated by any physical activity. High carbohydrate diets and fluid pills (diuretics) will usually help. Another symptom frequently encountered by high altitude runners is called a scin-

tillating scotomata. Flashing lights appear before the eyes
and are often accompanied by blurred vision, headache and
dizziness.

Ultraviolet rays of the sun are a great hazard to runners. This
topic is fully discussed in Chapter 12.

Pollution

Automobiles and air pollution are also important causes of
illness. Carbon monoxide, a chief component of automobile ex-
haust, binds tightly to red blood cells, preventing their normal
oxygen-carrying abilities. It may take several hours for carbon
monoxide to leave a runner's body. Therefore, running along
traffic-congested roads will decrease a runner's oxygen-carrying
capacity for at least one day. This problem can even cause more
acute illness. Recently a lead runner in South America stayed
too close to the official race car and collapsed from carbon monoxide poisoning.

Nighttime Running

Many runners prefer nighttime running. It is a good way to
avoid the extreme heat during summer. Be on the lookout, however, for potholes and other obstacles in the dark. In addition,
cars are a particular hazard at night, and reflective clothing
should be worn at all times. Always run against traffic during
the night, or avoid these problems by running on a track where
moonlight is usually sufficient for nighttime visibility.

An intelligent runner should carefully analyze the terrain and
environmental conditions when he plans his workout. Common
sense dictates that one does not run 20 miles on a track or do
speed work on a narrow rock-strewn wooded trail.

Automobiles

Day or night, cars are perhaps the greatest danger to a runner's
life. These mechanical monsters are runners' natural adversaries.
Unfortunately, arguing with a car is always a losing proposition.
Remember the basic principles: Always run against traffic; wear

reflective or brightly colored clothing under poor visibility conditions; avoid congested roads; and never trust an automobile driver. Always anticipate the worst and be prepared to step off the side of the road quickly if a car suddenly veers in your direction. A good trick is to watch the front tires of a car. This practice will give a few extra moments advance warning if a car suddenly swerves.

Assault, Rape and Robbery

While this may not be considered a major problem yet, as the popularity of running has increased over the past few years, so, unfortunately, has the incidence of assaults on runners. Most of these despicable incidents are perpetrated on women running alone in isolated areas. The best solution to this problem is prevention. A runner cannot always depend on his or her fleetness of foot to elude a criminal. Therefore, avoid running alone in deserted areas or at night; avoid "bad" neighborhoods; try to run with a companion; and cross the street or turn around when suspicious characters are lurking ahead. Weapons such as hatpins, tear gas and mace are of dubious value since they may be turned against the runner if seized by a strong assailant. A runner should always notify the police of suspicious persons, particularly those who make obscene comments. An official warning frequently prevents a budding lunatic from becoming a full-blown rapist.

Dogs

Many runners consider themselves former dog lovers. We all have our special stories of close encounters with the neighborhood Doberman pinscher. Yelling or making menacing gestures at dogs often dissuades them. Some runners carry small sticks, rocks, collapsed automobile radio antennas, water pistols filled with ammonia, tear gas, mace and other elements to ward off dogs. Unfortunately, these precautions are frequently necessary.

All dog bites should be reported to appropriate authorities. A pet should not be allowed to chase and bite runners. Remember, an unrestrained dog reflects a negligent owner. A concerted effort on the part of runners to prosecute owners to the full extent of the law is the only long-range solution to this growing problem.

Bee Stings

Bee stings are a life-threatening hazard to certain allergic runners (see Chapter 20).

MINOR INJURIES

A good runner is highly tuned to his body signals. Most major injuries are preceded by warning signs such as fatigue, muscle soreness, loss of appetite and insomnia, which often indicate that training loads have become too heavy. These symptoms usually improve after a day or so of light workouts or rest. By paying careful attention to other more specific minor injuries, such as nagging aches and pains, most major injuries that are preceded by these minor symptoms can usually be avoided. Never ignore pain during a workout. Many injuries begin with small tears of the muscle or tendon that gradually enlarge during further stress and exercise. If you note pain in a muscle or joint, immediately stop running and assess the situation. If the discomfort does not disappear after a few moments of rest, light stretching and easy jogging, discontinue the workout. The runner who insists on pushing himself with pain is actually hurting his training process. It is better to lighten workouts for a few days than to miss several months of training because of serious injury. In addition to application of ice, treatment includes rest, compression and elevation of the injured extremity (see Chapter 3.) Avoid measures that promote blood flow, such as heat and vigorous exercise. If a minor injury is properly treated, you can usually resume light running in 48 hours.

3

Treating Injuries

All runners develop injuries at some time or another, but with proper treatment these problems will not interfere with his long-range career. As stressed in the previous chapter, one of the common causes of serious injury is neglecting minor problems. A runner must listen to his body and take appropriate steps when injuries develop. There are five basic steps in the treatment of injuries:

- Immediate therapy to minimize damage
- Assessment of damage
- Assessment of cause
- Healing of injury
- Rehabilitation

IMMEDIATE TREATMENT

One of the most important measures that a runner can take to prevent disability is to minimize the degree of damage that occurs following an injury. Many injuries are associated with the rupture of small blood vessels, which causes bleeding into the tissues. In addition, the general inflammatory reaction following in injury causes fluid to leak out of blood vessels into the surrounding tissue. As a result of these processes, swelling develops during the first hour after an injury. The swelling stretches normal structures, resulting in pain and limitation of motion. In many instances damage that results from swelling can be worse than the initial injury. Blood and fluid may remain in the tissues long after an injury heals. Therefore, all injuries to the legs should be treated with measures aimed at minimizing tissue swelling.

Stop running. Never attempt to "run off" an injury. Running increases blood flow to the legs, thereby increasing the degree of swelling resulting from an injury. Even if an injury appears relatively mild, always assume the worst and stop running in order to minimize the degree of disability.

Elevate the leg above the level of the hip. This helps promote drainage of fluid from the leg into the rest of the body, thereby minimizing swelling. An injured extremity should be elevated on a pillow or blanket as quickly as possible.

Apply a compression wrap. Wrap injured areas with an elastic bandage in order to limit the degree of swelling. Specific wraps for injuries to the different areas of the body are described in the specific chapters dealing with those regions. Compression wraps should be snug, but never so tight that they interfere with circulation.

Finally, treat with a local ice pack. It is essential to minimize the degree of swelling. Cooling of the injured area minimizes inflammation and helps control bleeding. To prevent frostbite, apply ice packs over an elastic wrap intermittently, 20 minutes on, 10 minutes off. Repeat the application several times during the first 48 hours after an injury.

The sooner initial therapy of the injury is started, the greater the chances of minimizing subsequent disability. Elevation of the leg, compression wrap and ice packs should be continued for 1–2 hours after the initial injury. Then reassess the injury.

ASSESSMENT OF DAMAGE

A runner should be able to evaluate the degree of injury. Is there local swelling? Is there local heat or redness of the skin indicating inflammation or possible infection? Black, blue or yellow discoloration of the skin is a sign of local bleeding into the muscle or soft tissues, indicating a bruise, and may develop at any time from an hour to a few days after an injury. Is the local area tender? Often the injured structure can be identified by the exact location of pain and tenderness. A crunching or grinding of the tissue may indicate inflammation of a tendon or ligament. Inability to move a joint through its normal range of motion, or inability to bear weight on a leg may indicate a serious injury.

ASSESSING THE CAUSE OF AN INJURY

A runner must be able to assess the cause of his injury accurately. He should try to recall the exact sequence of events that caused the injury. Did he step into a pothole or twist his ankle on a rock? Did the injury develop suddenly with immediate pain and inability to run, or did his symptoms develop gradually over a period of several days?

In some instances the cause of an injury is obvious. In other cases a runner must think carefully to determine the cause of his problem. Pinpointing the cause of an injury can help to avoid recurrent problems. In addition, this information helps a doctor to evaluate and treat an injury.

One of the most common causes of injuries is overuse. Runners who push their bodies too far, too fast, exceeding the limits of their capabilities develop overuse injuries. They appear soon after a runner increases his weekly mileage or pushes himself too far in a race or a speed workout. Many runners are injured because they neglected one of the six basic principles discussed in Chapter 2. Refer to them and try to pinpoint the cause of an injury. The most common problems are: overuse, changing from one surface to another, breakdown from too much racing, improperly fitted or maintained shoes, and improper warm-up.

HEALING OF INJURIES

Severe injuries, particularly those that are incapacitating, should be brought to the immediate attention of a doctor. Otherwise, treat most injuries with rest, compression wrap and ice for the first 48 hours. We believe that early mobilization is an important element of proper healing and rehabilitation. After the initial 48 hours of rest and ice treatment, begin walking and then slow jogging as tolerated. After these workouts, reapply ice packs for at least 30 minutes to an hour. Depending upon the severity of the injury, this regimen of mobilization followed by ice followed by mobilization, and so on should continue for several days. If pain and swelling recur, start again, resting and reinstituting compression wraps and local ice therapy.

For 48–72 hours after an injury, anti-inflammatory medication is particularly useful to minimize pain and inflammation. Aspirin is an excellent drug for this purpose. Four to six aspirin tablets a day with two tablets taken a half hour before a workout are usually recommended. Be warned that aspirin does cause aggravation of peptic ulcer disease and can occasionally lead to gastrointestinal bleeding. It should be used with caution by people who have a history of peptic ulcers or other gastrointestinal problems. Nausea, abdominal pain, black stools and ringing in the ears are signals to stop taking aspirin and consult a doctor. Other over-the-counter pain relievers don't possess adequate anti-inflammatory action. Runners who can't take aspirin will require a prescription anti-inflammatory drug from their doctors. Runners who take aspirin should have their blood count checked periodically to detect insidious gastrointestinal blood loss.

Following a few days of ice and very light exercise, apply local heat for 15–20 minutes before a workout to help increase blood flow to an injured area and reduce pain during running. Various ways of applying local heat are described in a later section of this chapter. After a workout, however, ice should be applied to cool down the area quickly.

REHABILITATION

The purpose of rehabilitation is to restore the body to preinjury status and minimize the chances of recurrent injury. A well-structured, supervised rehabilitation program is essential for recovery from a disabling injury. Running ability is lost very quickly following an injury, especially when a joint or leg must be immobilized. Loss of ability starts after 2–3 days of immobilization. It takes about 3 days of rehabilitation to recover for every day lost to injury. After an injury, you can expect:

- Atrophy or loss of muscle size
- Loss of strength
- Loss of endurance
- Loss of flexibility
- Loss of coordination
- Loss of mental confidence

All of these lost functions must be properly treated to gain 100 percent recovery. Rehabilitation exercise programs should be started as soon as possible after an injury. This activity must be professionally supervised in order to insure the proper balance between exercise rehabilitation on one hand and the rest necessary for healing the injury on the other.

Normal range of motion and flexibility are the most difficult skills to restore. Prolonged disuse causes loss of elastic properties of structures around joints, sometimes producing permanent loss of full range of motion. Strength may be regained at any time, range of motion cannot. Therefore, quite early in a rehabilitation program each joint of an injured extremity should be moved through its complete range of motion. This can be done actively with a runner's own muscles, or if necessary, passively by a physical therapist or trainer. Note that when one structure of a leg is injured, all the other structures of that extremity also suffer. For example, when an ankle is immobilized for several weeks, the leg cannot be used properly, resulting in atrophy and loss of strength not only of the muscles surrounding the ankle, but also of the rest of the leg and thigh muscles. This fact must be taken into consideration when planning a rehabilitation program. If rehabilitation is aimed only at the injured ankle, it is likely that an injury to the thigh muscles on that same side will occur because of weakness and imbalance of those structures. For this reason, it is necessary to institute a generalized exercise program for all the muscles of an injured extremity in order to minimize the degree of atrophy and loss of strength.

Exercises include active and passive range of motion, isometric exercises, muscle stimulator therapy and weight training. Isometric exercises consist of moving a muscle against an immovable object. For example, a quadriceps isometric exercise consists of sitting in a chair with legs under a heavy desk and pushing up with thighs trying to lift desk. An adductor muscle isometric exercise consists of lying on the floor and trying to squeeze a pillow placed between the thighs. Contractions should be held for approximately 6–10 seconds, and programs usually start with sets of 5–10 repetitions. Muscle stimulator machines are devices that cause muscles to contract by stimulating them with an electric current. This device is relatively painless and quite effective. Specific weight-training exercises for each muscle region are illustrated in Figure 3-1. Injured athletes should engage in a graduated muscle-strengthening program consisting of one or all of these methods until they have regained normal strength. Initial therapy should generally start with two daily sessions of muscle-strengthening exercises. Once intensive weight strengthening begins, sessions may be performed once a day or every other day. In addition to muscle strengthening, specific exercises to help recover from various injuries are described in the particular chapters dealing with those injuries.

Cardiovascular fitness and endurance can be maintained during rehabilitation by substitute exercises such as swimming, rowing or bicycling. Most injured runners prefer swimming, which can be performed even while wearing a lightweight waterproof leg cast.

In addition to muscle-strengthening exercises, cold, heat, ultrasonic vibration and massage are used to treat injured athletes. Different physicians and trainers may prefer one to another, but they are all valid as part of a rehabilitation program.

Cold

As previously discussed, local application of ice is the first treatment for acute minor injury. This can be accomplished safely either with ice cubes packed in plastic bags or with the use of commercially available chemical cold packs. Chemical cold packs can be purchased at sporting goods stores and are

muscle-strengthening exercises

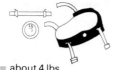

bar = about 4 lbs
discs = 2½ lbs, 5 lbs
Total maximum = 45 lbs

suggested equipment

Use an iron boot weighing about 5 lbs.
Strap to foot.
To add weight, insert iron bar in hole.
Add circles as tolerated.
Tighten cuffs on bar so that they are secure.

1. quadriceps exercise 3 x 10

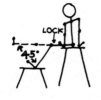

1. Fully extend leg.
2. Lock knee - bring toe up.
3. Hold for count of 3.
4. Lower slowly.
5. Repeat 30 times, resting after each set of 10.

note: Do not exceed 15 lbs without permission.
Increase weight about 1 lb a day. At 25 lbs, activity (e.g.
running, swimming, dancing) may be added. At 45 lbs, can
resume full activity.

note: Never let foot hang straight; always lift from 45°
or less.

2. hip flexor 3 x 10

1. Lie flat on back on floor or firm table.
2. Raise your leg straight up, knee stiff.
3. Hold.
4. Bring it down slowly.
5. Repeat 30 times, resting after each set of 10.

note: Do not exceed 15 lbs without permission.

3. abduction and adduction 3 x 10

1. Lie flat on back on floor or firm table.
2. Raise foot up 12 inches.
3. Spread leg to side.
4. Return to center, then down to original position.
5. Repeat 30 times, resting after each set of 10.

note: Do not exceed 15 lbs without permission.

4. hamstring

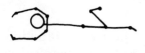

1. Lie on front on floor or firm table.
2. Bring heel to buttocks.
3. Slowly lower.
4. Repeat 30 times, resting after each set of 10.

note: Do not exceed 15 lbs without permission. If necessary a rolled towel under knee will lessen pressure on
knee cap.

Figure 3-1

usually used for convenience when ice is not available. They remain cold for about 30 minutes and, like ice packs, should not be applied directly to the skin. We recommend an initial period of local application for 15–30 minutes. Reapply the pack several times during the subsequent 48 hours. Do not apply cold by immersing the injured limb in ice buckets, which is not only uncomfortable but may also lead to frostbite. In addition, an immersed limb hangs downward, thus increasing swelling.

Heat

Local heat is frequently recommended for the late treatment of acute injuries and can be applied in any of the following ways:

HYDROCOLATORS

A hydrocolator steam pack is an excellent method of applying local heat. This device is a cloth bag divided into compartments containing a special gel filler that absorbs water. When heated it retains warmth for a long period of time. The pack is warmed in a pot of water, wrapped in a hot towel, then applied to the injured area. Be careful not to burn yourself when using one. They may be purchased at surgical supply houses and many drugstores.

ELECTRIC HEAT PADS

Electric heat pads heat through conductivity when in contact with the body. They are particularly useful when heat is required for long periods of time. These pads should be enclosed in a towel in order to promote perspiration and local moist heat. Runners should use only waterproof heating pads to prevent electric shocks. Don't fall asleep with a heating pad as severe burns may result.

DIATHERMY

A diathermy is a machine that produces shortwave radiation. This device produces deep heat in injured muscles and is frequently helpful in treating deep injuries that do not respond to hydrocolators or heat pads.

HEAT LAMPS

Heat lamps provide convective heat. The radiant-type heat lamp is usually preferable. It has a tungsten filament bulb which is enclosed in a reflector and produces heat that will penetrate up to ⅜ inch beneath the skin and will dilate local blood vessels, thereby increasing blood flow to an injured area. Treatment sessions should last for approximately 30 minutes. To prevent burns, do not place the lamp too close to the skin. Applying oil to the skin improves the results of treatment and also helps prevent burns. Ultaviolet lamps are not recommended because of the adverse effects of ultraviolet light.

WHIRLPOOL BATHS

Whirlpool baths combine moist heat with gentle water massage. The water should be between 106°–110° F, and therapy should last for approximately 20 minutes. Using a whirlpool bath too early in the course of treatment may lead to hemorrhage and swelling of the dependent limb. Therefore, these treatments are usually reserved for later phases of injury treatment and may be combined with exercise therapy.

HOT BATHS

Many runners enjoy hot baths after a workout. These may be simple bathtubs or elaborate Jacuzzi baths. The temperature of the water should start at 98° F and be gradually increased to 105° F, and should be limited to 30 minutes since severe exhaustion and sweat loss can result from longer immersion.

CONTRAST BATHS

Contrast baths are used to treat sprains and contusions by increasing blood flow to the injured area. The injured extremity is immersed in hot water (100°–110° F) for 3 minutes, then cold water (50°–65° F) for 1 minute. The process is repeated five times, ending with the hot water bath.

LINIMENTS AND BALMS

Liniments and balms are used to relieve pain and bring local heat to a sore muscle. Their basic ingredients are menthyl salicylate (oil of wintergreen), oil of turpentine, oil of capsicum (red pepper), camphor, oil of mustard and many other varieties. These substances are mixed either in a light oil base to produce liniments or in a heavy petroleum substance to make balms. These agents cause local irritation which stimulates nerves and increases local blood flow. They produce redness and warmth of the skin, but their value is questionable since they probably don't penetrate very deeply beneath the skin.

In general, apply a liniment or balm prior to a workout and wash it off afterward to prevent excessive skin irritation. Occasionally, hot packs are devised using balms or ointments. The ointment is applied to the skin and the area is covered with cotton and wrapped with an elastic bandage (Figure 3-2). Once again, this hot pack is to be used only during a workout and not to be worn for extended periods of time.

Ultrasonic Vibrators

Ultrasonic vibrators produce energy in the form of vibrations occurring at between a hundred thousand and a million vibrations per second. This high frequency sound produces an effect in tissues similar to deep heat. Use this techinque only under professional supervision as improper use can result in tissue damage.

Massage

Massage is the scientific and systematic manipulation of tissue for therapeutic purposes. When done properly, massage will increase circulation and promote drainage of an injured area. There are three types of medical massage: stroking, kneading and friction.

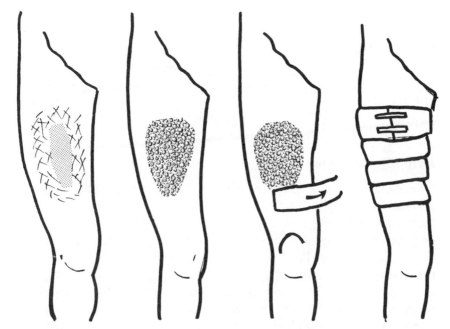

Apply balm or liniment to skin, cover with cotton and wrap with an elastic bandage. Wash agents off skin after workout.

Figure 3-2 HOT PACK FOR SORE MUSCLES

The basic stroking technique consists of long sweeping movements along the contours of the body, applied with the palm of the hand directly on the skin, using a firm and even motion. The pressure may be light or deep. The deeper the pressure, the deeper the massage. Kneading consists of wringing the tissues by lifting, rolling or squeezing. A friction massage is performed with deep circular rolling movements, using the tips of the fingers and the palms of the hands. This technique is helpful for breaking down small scars and loosening stiff joints and sore muscles.

Massage should start with stroking. Kneading and friction massage may then follow. Start from the end of a limb and direct massage toward the heart. Lubricants are generally employed. Hairy skin requires larger amounts of lubricant. Mineral oil, cocoa butter, olive oil, petroleum jelly or talcum powder may be used.

EQUIPMENT

In order to care for minor injuries properly, a runner should have some basic equipment on hand. A suggested runner's first aid kit is shown in Table 3-1. In addition, certain items that require further explanation are listed here.

Adhesive or Chiropodist Felt

A versatile item used for the treatment of various injuries, adhesive or chiropodist felt is available in thicknesses varying from ⅟₁₆ to ½ inch. Its cushioning properties are used to relieve pressure on an irritated or inflamed structure. A felt pad should be used around, and not on top of the affected area. This bridging principle distributes weight away from an inflamed area. For example, donut-shaped pads are used around the margins of blisters (Chapter 12), and felt tracks on each side of an inflamed tendon (Chapter 5). These pads absorb the pressure and friction of shoes and permit running without irritation. A piece of felt placed inside each shoe also acts as an arch support (Chapter 5).

TABLE 3-1

Runner's First Aid Kit

Petroleum jelly	Ice bags
Moleskin	Corn and callus file
Adhesive felt	Safety pins
Band-Aids	Iodine antiseptic
Gauze pads	Antibiotic ointment (Neosporin)
70% rubbing alcohol	Antifungal powder and cream
Hydrocolator pack or heating pad	(Desenex, Tinactin)
Scissor	Sunscreen lotion
Nail clipper	Analgesic balm
Elastic bandages	Aspirin
Adhesive tape	Antacids (Maalox, Gelusil)
Thermometer	Skin softener for calluses (Nivea
Talcum powder	cream)

Moleskin

Moleskin is an adhesive pad that is thinner than chiropodist felt, but much thicker than normal adhesive tape to give it a padding effect when used to cover sensitive areas of skin. It very effectively protects feet from painful shoe pinching and rubbing. Moleskin is often applied directly to "hot spots," sensitive areas of skin, before blisters develop. In addition, old blister spots may be covered with moleskin to prevent the development of new blisters. Moleskin, however, should never be used over recently broken blisters, cuts or lacerations. Once it is placed on a blister, it should be allowed to fall off by itself, for pulling it may tear the underlying skin.

Orthoplast

Orthoplast, a brand name for a semirigid plastic, is used for lightweight casts. It can be easily molded when heated with hot water and holds its form when it cools. It is very versatile—easy to cut, mold and fit. The perforated type of Orthoplast is very lightweight and makes excellent arch supports and splints.

Elastic (Ace) Bandages

Versatile elastic bandages may be used to support an injured joint, to apply compression to a damaged area or to hold an ice pack or a heating pad in place. Elastic bandages come in 2-, 3-, 4-, and 6-inch widths. Generally, a runner should base his choice of elastic bandage on the circumference of the area to be supported. Ankle sprains will require 2-inch bandages, while thigh compression wraps require 6-inch size. Ready-made elastic supports such as knee supports are generally inferior to properly applied roll-type elastic bandages.

Adhesive Tape

Adhesive tape is an essential item in any first aid cabinet. It has a wide variety of uses, from support of an injured joint or a broken toe and correction of an abnormal foot plant to stabilization of an arch support or felt pad. The most common width used in athletic treatment is 1½ inches. This size will fit most of the contours of the feet and knees. As most of us know, adhesive tape that adheres to hair is painful to remove. To avoid this discomfort, shave the skin area before covering it with tape. A lightweight underwrap material between skin and tape further protects skin from damage when the tape is removed. Runners with sensitive skin may wish to use nonallergic paper tape, although its adhesive properties are not quite as strong as the cloth type.

Heel Cups

Heel cups are used to protect bruised heels as well as to minimize the irritation of bone spurs of the heel. They are made of unbreakable plastic and come in one size only. With body heat, the cup molds to the heel and forms a firm supporting structure. Heel cups also help prevent blisters, hot spots and local areas of irritation from forming on the skin of the heel.

4

Basic Injuries

The vast majority of runners' injuries occur to those structures below the waist that are used during the motion of running. From the ground up, these areas are: the foot, ankle, leg, knee, thigh, hip and back. You will better understand the problems involving each one after a brief review of the basic structure of the body's tissues and the mechanisms by which injuries occur.

The tissues that usually sustain injuries during running are: muscles, bones, tendons, ligaments, joints, bursa and fascia. By understanding how each of these different tissues can be injured, a runner can apply that information to specific anatomical regions. Most runners' injuries can be classified as follows:

• *A direct blow (trauma, contusion)*. This type of injury can affect several tissues at the same time. Broken blood vessels usually cause local bleeding and swelling of the injured tissues. Examples: a kick in the leg, running into an object.

• *A tear or rupture (pull, strain)*. This injury usually involves muscles or tendons and may vary from a microscopic tear to a complete rupture of the structure. Example: a muscle tear or tendon rupture sustained during strenuous running.

• *Inflammation*. This may involve any type of tissue. It is usually secondary to irritation or overuse. Local tenderness and swelling of the tissue are often present. Example: tendinitis and myositis—inflammation of tendon and muscle respectively—can follow an overdose of speed work.

• *A partial or complete break (fracture)*. Bone may be fractured from a direct blow or from overuse. Example: a stress fracture of the metatarsal bones in the foot from training at distances beyond your capacity.

• *Sprain (overstretching)*. Ligaments may be sprained from stumbling or twisting a joint. Example: an ankle sprain from stumbling in a pothole.

• *Infection*. The cause of infection is invasion and irritation of tissue by bacteria, viruses or sometimes fungi. Example: osteomyelitis—a bacterial infection of bone—can be one result of a deep puncture wound.

Each of these different types of injury will be discussed in relation to the different types of tissues.

One type of injury that may involve several types of tissues is an overuse injury which, as the term implies, occurs when a runner overextends himself, pushing too far, too quickly. It takes time for the body to adapt to the exertion of running. High mileage and speed training require increased demands on a runner's tissues, and it takes time for these structures to adapt by becoming larger and stronger during training. The overuse syndrome describes those injuries which result from high mileage training, speed work or changing from a soft to a hard running surface. Overuse injuries can involve any body tissue, resulting in inflammation, strain, stress fracture and occasionally, more serious injury.

MUSCLE TISSUE

Basic Structure and Function

Muscle is a specialized tissue composed of protein filaments that slide over each other to produce muscle contraction (Figure 4-1). Power for this process comes from conversion of chemical energy into kinetic or movement energy. Energy for muscle contraction is supplied by a high energy molecule called adeno-

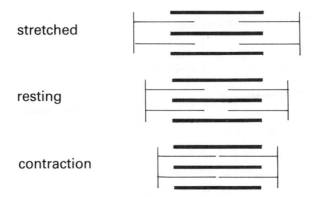

stretched

resting

contraction

Muscle cells are composed of protein filaments that slide over each other to enable muscle to stretch and contract during exercise.

Figure 4-1.   MUSCLE STRUCTURE

sine triphosphate (ATP), which is produced in the muscle from metabolism of carbohydrates and fats. During endurance-type exercise, such as long distance running, ATP is continually re-made by a chemical reaction using oxygen, carbohydrates and fats. This process, called oxidative metabolism, is the biochemical equivalent to aerobic exercise. On the other hand, sprinting and weight lifting require short bursts of muscle contraction and are performed without consumption of oxygen. This anoxidative metabolism produces ATP molecules for short-term exercise and is the equivalent of anaerobic exercise. Anaerobic energy production can last for only 2–3 minutes, after which an accumulation of lactic acid and an oxygen debt preclude continued activity.

There are two predominant types of muscle cells. Type I (light, fast twitch or phasic muscle fibers) contract quickly and derive energy from anoxidative metabolism. They provide rapid movements for a relatively short period of time and are used for sprinting. Type II (dark, slow twitch or tonic muscle fibers) have a slower contraction speed. They use oxidative metabolism and function during prolonged activity, such as distance running.

All human muscles have a mixture of both types of muscle fibers. Some muscles which are used mainly for fast movements have a slight predominance of fast twitch fibers, while those used for prolonged activity such as standing (the antigravity muscles) have a slight predominance of slow twitch fibers. The percentage of fast and slow twitch fibers present in each individual runner is, to a large extent, genetically determined.

Training Effects

Training enables muscles to become more efficient in the production of ATP during exercise. The necessary enzymes within muscle cells will increase approximately twofold. Endurance training increases those used for oxidative production of ATP, while sprinting and anaerobic training will increase enzymes used for anoxidative metabolism. Endurance training also increases the number of slow twitch muscle fibers, and sprint training and speed work increase the number of fast twitch muscle fibers in running muscles. Muscle fiber composition can be influenced to some extent by training, but it is still uncertain what percentage of fast and slow twitch fibers is genetically determined and what percentage can be altered by training.

Training also strengthens the cardiovascular system which then supplies increased oxygen to exercising muscles. Alterations include increased cardiac output by a trained runner's heart and increased blood vessel supply to exercising muscle. (See Chapter 15 for further discussion of cardiovascular changes with training.)

The length of time spent on each workout will affect these training adaptations. Studies indicate that increased blood vessel supply to exercising muscle develops much quicker when muscle is continually exercised for 2 or more hours. Enzymatic alterations also seem to be maximized by runs of this duration. It takes about 6 weeks of training for these enzyme changes to occur.

Training stimulates enzymes that burn fats rather than carbohydrates. As previously discussed, oxidative metabolism can use either carbohydrate or fat as fuel for production of ATP. Carbohydrate is generally the preferred fuel and is used preferentially during the first 2 hours of running. However, after that time or approximately 20 miles of running, muscle is depleted of carbohydrate and must switch to fat as fuel. This carbohydrate depletion is thought to represent one of the major factors producing the so-called "wall phenomenon" sometimes experienced during the last miles of a marathon. Well-trained distance runners are able to utilize fat for oxidative metabolism more easily because they have a high number of enzymes necessary for the use of fat as fuel. Their muscles are able to burn fat during the early phases of long distance runs and the switch-over from carbohydrate to fatty metabolism does not produce such an abrupt collapse. Ultramarathoners primarily burn fat as running fuel. According to a recent discovery, caffeine helps induce or stimulate those enzymes which burn fat. Runners who take caffeine equivalent to two cups of coffee one hour before a race are able to burn fat much more efficiently and may gain a competitive advantage in races over 5,000 kilometers.

Muscle Injuries

Much of the terminology regarding muscle injuries is confusing. Pulled muscle, torn muscle, charley horse, cramp, and so on are often used indiscriminately. To avoid confusion, a runner should understand the basic types of muscle injuries and apply this knowledge to the particular muscle group in question. To avoid repetition, the causes and basic treatment of each of these types of injuries are detailed in this chapter, and the runner should refer to this section in later chapters that deal with specific muscles.

The basic muscle injuries are: muscle strain, muscle rupture, muscle spasm, myositis, painful muscle scar, muscle atrophy, muscle contusion and myositis ossificans (Figure 4-2).

MUSCLE STRAIN

Cause: Muscle strain or muscle pull represents a partial tear of a muscle and is usually caused by overuse or excessive stress. This injury can occur gradually during several consecutive days of high mileage, or it can be an acute injury developing during speed work or a race. Muscle strains are much more common among runners who do not perform proper warm-up and stretching exercises.

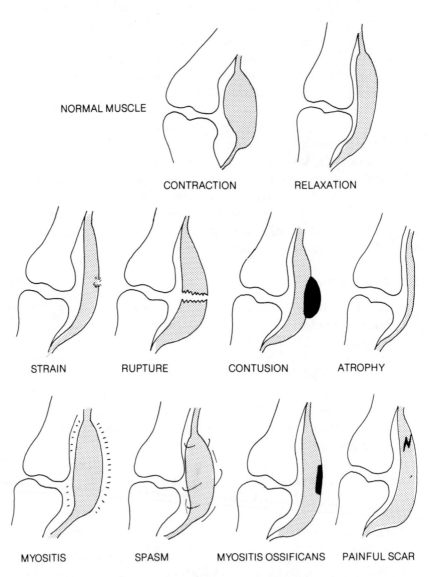

NORMAL MUSCLE

CONTRACTION RELAXATION

STRAIN RUPTURE CONTUSION ATROPHY

MYOSITIS SPASM MYOSITIS OSSIFICANS PAINFUL SCAR

Figure 4-2. MUSCLE INJURIES

The muscle injury is often associated with local blood vessel damage resulting in leakage of fluid and blood into the surrounding muscle which, in turn, causes tissue swelling. In addition, the injured muscle can develop spasm which produces local pain and tenderness.

Symptoms and Diagnosis: Symptoms may be gradual or sudden, depending upon the manner of the injury. Injuries associated with muscle spasm are usually painful. A minor strain can produce mild pain several hours after a workout, while a larger tear can cause a sprinter suddenly to pull up lame in the middle of the race. Swelling and local tenderness are often present. When muscle spasm is a major component, the muscle will feel very firm to the touch.

Mild cases of muscle strain must be differentiated from myositis and from hot weather muscle cramps. Since myositis and muscle cramps usually disappear within a relatively short time, persistent pain in a muscle suggests a muscle strain.

More severe muscle tears are usually easily diagnosed by the circumstance of the injury and the location of the pain.

Comments and Treatment: Treat muscle strains as quickly as possible. To minimize local bleeding and swelling of the muscle, immediately stop running and apply compression and ice packs to the injured muscle. It is best to restrict activities until the bleeding has totally stopped—a period of between 24–48 hours. If walking and light jogging cause no pain at this point, gradually resume a training schedule. But proceed *slowly*, since small tears can turn into more serious problems.

Most small muscle strains heal within 2 weeks, at which time regular training schedules can be resumed, although racing and hard workouts should generally be postponed for 3–4 weeks.

MUSCLE RUPTURE

Cause: Occasionally a muscle is so severely injured that it completely ruptures. Muscles most commonly involved are the rectus femoris of the quadriceps, the hamstrings—especially the biceps femoris, and the gastrocnemius and soleus muscles of the calf. Runners develop ruptured muscles in much the same way that partial tears or strains occur.

Symptoms and Diagnosis: A complete muscle tear causes the dramatic onset of severe pain in the involved muscle. Spasm of muscle is usual, resulting in a bulge. The injury produces exquisite pain and inability to run or move the muscle through its normal range of motion.

The location of the pain usually helps to distinguish a muscle rupture from a ruptured tendon. Since muscle rupture is a severe condition, a runner should seek immediate medical attention if this type of injury occurs.

Comments and Treatment: Treatment of a muscle rupture depends upon the muscle involved and the location of the injury. In some cases when a muscle has ruptured near the place of its insertion to the bone, surgical repair is attempted. In other instances, surgery offers no benefit. Whatever the case, this is one injury that must be treated by a physician.

Atrophy (discussed later in chapter) and muscle weakness almost always follow muscle rupture. Therefore, before returning to full activity, a runner needs an exercise-strengthening regimen. In addition, a stretching program should begin during early rehabilitation to avoid muscle shortening due to scar tissue.

MUSCLE SPASM

Cause: Muscle spasm or muscle cramp is the sustained contraction of a muscle as a result of injury or other irritation. Some instances of muscle spasm result from overworking the muscles without significant injury. This type is most common during hot weather running, although the exact connection between the heat and muscle spasm is still uncertain. These so-called heat cramps are frequently attributed to salt depletion. In reality, however, they probably represent a combination of water and salt loss, coupled with minor muscle tear and injury. They may occur during or several hours after running. (See Hot Weather Diseases in Chapter 17.)

In other cases, a muscle spasm may signal a muscle tear or rupture and usually occurs within moments of the muscle injury.

Symptoms and Diagnosis: Muscle cramps cause severe local pain, tenderness and spasm of the involved muscle, which usually force a runner to stop. The sudden painful tightening of a muscle and the inability to relax it signals a muscle spasm.

Comments and Treatment: When a runner develops a muscle spasm, he should immediately stop running before the muscle becomes so tight that excruciating pain develops. It is imperative to stretch the muscle immediately and relieve the spasm. For example, a cramp of the calf muscle is treated by straightening the knee and bending the foot upward. After stretching, massage the involved area to relax the muscle and reduce pain.

If the muscle spasm and pain are rapidly relieved by stretching, it is safe to resume easy jogging. If the spasm recurs, however, then *muscle strain is likely,* and it is best to stop training and treat the strain.

MYOSITIS

Cause: Mild inflammation of muscle is called myositis or sore muscles. Myositis is caused by overuse of a group of muscles that have been pushed beyond their normal limits. It involves microscopic damage and swelling of the inflamed muscles. A long distance runner may develop sore muscles after an unusual speed workout, while a sprinter may develop sore muscles following an unaccustomed high mileage run. Myositis is a common complaint the day after a marathon.

Symptoms and Diagnosis: Diffuse aches and local tenderness develop in large muscle groups 24–48 hours after an unusually strenuous run. Runners who develop sore muscles are usually aware that they have pushed themselves beyond their limits. This problem can be differentiated from more serious problems, such as muscle strains or tendinitis, because myositis causes much more generalized muscle soreness and involves both legs.

Comments and Treatment: Myositis is a mild condition that improves within a few days. Contrary to most overuse injuries, myositis improves more quickly if running is not discontinued. Therefore, if a runner notes extreme soreness of his legs on the day following a long distance race, he should attempt an easy workout to help loosen his muscles. This may consist of an easy walk or a jog, depending on your individual abilities. Sometimes moist heat, such as a warm bath, may be necessary to decrease the pain prior to a workout. In addition, taking two aspirin tablets three or four times a day usually helps speed recovery from this condition.

Myositis represents inflammation of muscles that are pushed beyond their limits, and a training program should be structured to prevent this type of extreme stress. More severe injuries will occur if a runner repeatedly tries to exceed his abilities.

PAINFUL MUSCLE SCAR

Cause: Partial or complete muscle tears form scar tissue as they heal. Scar tissue is not elastic like muscle tissue, and as a result, tightness of muscles may develop. Running can stretch and reinjure tissue in the area of an old scar causing inflammation and pain. This process can become a vicious cycle as restretching and tearing an old scar causes inflammation and further scar formation, resulting in chronic muscle pain and disability.

Symptoms and Diagnosis: Pain and tenderness of a muscle around an old injury suggest inflammation of scar tissue. This pain can be aggravated by vigorous stretching and long runs which apply increased stress on the injured muscle. In addition, a runner will frequently note a lump and spasm of the involved muscle.

Comments and Treatment: The object of treatment is to decrease the inflammation and break the cycle of repeated injury and scar formation. Ease up on workouts and take aspirin for several days to allow the injury time to begin healing. Once the pain has diminished, start a gentle stretching program to allow use of the muscle without further injury to the scar mass. In some cases, treatment includes a physician or therapist using ultrasound and deep massage to break up the old scar tissue. Because a muscle that has significant scarring is often weak and atrophied, endurance training and muscle strengthening are essential parts of a treatment regimen.

MUSCLE ATROPHY

Cause: Muscle atrophy means loss of muscle size, although this term is sometimes applied to loss of muscle strength and endurance not necessarily associated with decreased muscle size. Atrophy is caused either by not using the muscle, or by injuring the nerves supplying the muscle. For example, thigh muscles will atrophy after a knee or ankle injury requiring immobilization of the whole leg, or after damaging the nerves that supply these muscles due to a slipped intravertebral disc.

Symptoms and Diagnosis: Most frequently, runners will note atrophy during recovery from an injury that caused temporary disuse of the involved muscles. Muscle atrophy is often obvious when a runner compares the muscle to the normal muscle of the other limb. In addition, weakness associated with muscle atrophy may cause instability around the knee and ankle joints.

Comments and Treatment: Muscle atrophy occurs *rapidly* following a period of inactivity or local injury. Before resuming a full training schedule, specific exercises are necessary to restore muscle strength to normal (see Chapter 3). Some runners mistakenly believe that running alone is adequate rehabilitation. Unfortunately, this is not the case, since the stresses being placed on atrophied muscles are often more than they can handle, and chronic imbalance and injury of the muscle or associated joints may occur. For this reason, any injury that requires partial or complete immobilization of a specific muscle group for more than a week should be treated with a muscle strengthening and endurance program. As a general rule of thumb, it takes 3 days of muscle strengthening exercises to make up for each day of muscle immobilization.

Muscle atrophy associated with nerve injuries is more complex and should be evaluated and treated by an orthopedic surgeon and/or a neurosurgeon.

MUSCLE BRUISE (CONTUSION)

Cause: A muscle bruise or contusion usually results from a local blow sustained by running into an object or falling and striking an area of muscle. Severe blows cause tear and rupture of small blood vessels within the muscle tissue resulting in bleeding and local blood clot. Once blood has escaped into the muscle tissue, it is a very painful irritant, causing accumulation of fluid and muscle spasm. The injured tissue itself usually heals long before the body is able to absorb the blood clot that has formed and which can severely interfere with running activities. The degree of limitation is directly related to the size of the clot.

Symptoms and Diagnosis: A runner will note pain, swelling and spasm following trauma to a muscle. As bleeding progresses, the swelling and discomfort increase, sometimes making running impossible. Most bruises are painful to some degree, but significant local swelling and inability to continue running suggest a large muscle contusion and a blood clot.

Comments and Treatment: This muscle injury cannot be "run out." In fact, continued running increases bleeding and only aggravates the problem. To minimize the bleeding as quickly as possible, treat relatively severe blows to a muscle by taking these steps:

- Stop running immediately.
- Apply a compression wrap such as an Ace bandage to decrease the local bleeding. It should be comfortable and snug but not so tight that it interferes with the blood supply to the rest of the leg.
- Apply an ice pack directly over the wrap in the area of the contusion.

After 2 or 3 hours, reassess the severity of the injury. If the bruise appears relatively mild, attempt easy walking. Be cautious, however, for the first 2 days to prevent further bleeding.

If there is severe local pain, tenderness and swelling after 2 or 3 hours, apply ice and compression for at least another 24 hours and rest. If you must walk, use crutches to keep the injured leg immobilized. The ideal treatment is bed rest with the leg elevated above chest level for the initial 24 hours. While ice packs can be discontinued after 48 hours, the compression wrap and limited activity should be the rule for several days. Increased pain or swelling means further bleeding, necessitating ice pack treatment for an additional 24 hours.

If 24–48 hours of ice and compression control the symptoms, resume light walking and progress to gradual jogging. If, however, soreness and pain with movement continue, seek medical help. After 3–4 days of additional rest, local moist heat may speed the blood clot resorption, but overtreatment such as massage, deep heat and muscle injections can aggravate the condition.

If it takes several days to recover from a muscle bruise, a certain amount of muscle atrophy has probably occurred and must be treated with muscle strengthening and rehabilitation before you resume running.

CHARLEY HORSE

At the old Ebbets Field of the Brooklyn Dodgers, there was a horse who pulled a piece of chain-link fence around the infield between innings. As the years passed, the horse grew quite lame and developed a significant limp. The horse's name was Charley, and since that time any athletic injury that produces lameness has been referred to as a "charley horse." According to correct athletic medicine nomenclature, the term charley horse means muscle contusion. Athletes, however, continue to apply the term loosely to various injuries from tendinitis to muscle strains, tears and contusions. To avoid confusion, it is best to strike charley horse from your vocabulary altogether.

MYOSITIS OSSIFICANS

Cause: For reasons that are not completely clear, myositis ossificans (calcification or bone formation) sometimes occurs within an area of muscle following a severe contusion. The front and side of the thighs are most commonly involved. It is an unpredictable complication, not directly related to the severity of the injury. One runner may develop myositis ossificans, while another with an equally severe injury may not.

Symptoms and Diagnosis: Increased pain, tenderness and heat occurring a few days after a muscle contusion, as well as muscle spasm and inability to extend or flex the involved muscle, indicate myositis ossificans. X rays will also show bony changes in the muscle 2–3 weeks after injury.

Comments and Treatment: Proper treatment of muscle contusion usually prevents myositis ossificans, but once it occurs, it is a serious complication which must be treated by an experienced physician.

Restrict activity to a level that can be maintained without local pain. The best treatment is an initial "cooling off" rest period. After several weeks, resume a gradual schedule of strengthening and endurance exercises, followed by full running activity to assess the degree of disability.

Avoid any type of local manipulation such as massage, heat, ultrasound and injections, which may aggravate myositis ossificans. When the amount of bone formed within the muscle restricts activity, surgical removal may be necessary. This is best performed 6 months to a year after the initial injury.

BONE

Basic Structure

Bone supports and protects the human body and is essential for movement. Muscles move the body by pulling bones that surround joints. Bone consists of calcium phosphate which is a mineral that gives bone its hard consistency, and collagen which is a supporting tissue that binds other tissues together. In addition to forming a lattice work upon which the minerals of bone are deposited, collagen adds resiliency and shock-absorbing capacity to bony structures. Bone is covered by a thin tissue called periosteum which contains nerve fibers and blood vessels.

Training Adaptations

When bone is subjected to stress over a period of months, it will adjust by remodeling itself so that it is stronger in the area of the greatest stress. The bones of runners, therefore, are usually stronger and denser in those regions where tendons from leg muscles attach to the bone. Changes, however, take months to occur for, of all the body's tissues, bone takes the longest to adapt to stress. Many beginning runners who have quickly developed cardiovascular and muscular fitness develop bone injuries such as stress fractures because their bones have not yet adjusted to the increased stresses of training.

Bone Injuries

There are four main bone injuries that runners may develop: stress fracture, periostitis, bone bruise and complete bone fracture.

STRESS FRACTURE

Cause: Stress fracture is an overuse injury which results in a partial break in the surface of a bone. The most common site of runners' stress fractures are the end of the tibia (leg) bone near the ankle and the metatarsal bones of the foot. Runners occasionally develop stress fractures of the neck of the femur (thigh) bone.

This injury appears to develop because excessive stress is placed on bone before it has adapted to training. Most commonly, stress fractures develop after high mileage training or switching to a harder running surface.

Symptoms and Diagnosis: Pain occurs gradually in the area of damaged bone. Local tenderness and slight swelling may be noted. Symptoms increase during running and eventually become chronic. Then, pain is present during walking, weight bearing or movement of the extremity. Elevation of the leg usually relieves the symptoms.

Persistent pain in one area of bone, particularly over the end of the tibia or the metatarsal bones, suggests a stress fracture. After 2–3 weeks, stress fractures can usually be seen on X rays as small breaks in the outer margin of the bone. However, X rays taken within the first 2 weeks of an injury will *not* show abnormalities. A bone scan is a more sensitive indicator of bone damage and may be performed if the pain is severe. A small amount of radioactive substance (radioisotope) is injected into the bloodstream. The isotope localizes in areas of injured bone and is detected by a sophisticated Geiger counter.

Comments and Treatment: The treatment of stress fracture depends upon the severity of the fracture and the bone involved. Stress fracture of a major weight-bearing bone such as a tibia or femur must be treated more conservatively than a fracture of a fibula, a relatively nonweight-bearing bone. An improperly treated stress fracture can progress to a complete break in the bone.

The initial treatment for stress fracture is to stop running and rest the injured extremity. Runners with stress fractures of weight-bearing bones must use crutches. Once the healing process begins, gradual weight bearing is usually allowed. This initial recovery period may take from 2–6 weeks. Since atrophy of muscles occurs rapidly following immobilization of an injured leg, strengthening exercises are an important part of the rehabilitation program.

This injury is a definite sign of overuse. To avoid recurrence, alter your training program and choose shoes that have excellent shock-absorbing properties of the sole. Try to run on soft surfaces such as grass and avoid hard surfaces such as roads and concrete, particularly during long mileage runs. By gradually strengthening bones, runners will be able eventually to tolerate high mileage running without difficulty. But this training adaptation of bones is a gradual process requiring several months, so plan your training program accordingly. (For further discussion, see individual chapters dealing with the specific stress fractures of the tibia, fibula, metatarsals and femur bones.)

PERIOSTITIS

Cause: Inflammation of the periosteum—thin tissue that surrounds bone—is called periostitis. Most authorities think that this injury is a precursor of stress fracture, and it usually results from the same overuse factors. This syndrome is one of the most common causes of shin splint pain as well as a common injury of runners with unusual running styles.

Symptoms and Diagnosis: Diffuse pain and swelling over the involved bone is usual. The pain increases during running and is relieved by rest. Periostitis is often bilateral (involves both legs). Because periostitis and stress fracture frequently represent different degrees of severity of the same injury, it is not always necessary to distinguish one from the other. Afflicted runners should see a physician so that X rays and bone scans can be considered (see Chapter 7 for discussion of shin splints).

Comments and Treatment: Periostitis should be treated early before it becomes a chronic condition and develops into stress fracture. When the symptoms become severe, take aspirin and apply local heat packs over an elastic bandage wrap. In addition, restrict running activity to soft-surface, low-mileage workouts until pain disappears. It is usually not necessary to stop running completely.

OSTEOMYELITIS

Infection of bone with bacteria is called osteomyelitis. Bacteria can travel through the bloodstream to lodge in bone and cause infection, and direct injury to bone such as a deep laceration or compound (open) fracture may cause contamination. Skin infections such as boils can cause spread of bacteria into the bloodstream and subsequent infection of bone, or a chronic toenail infection can cause osteomyelitis of the underlying bone. A deep puncture wound sustained while running barefoot can infect the bones of the foot. In addition, a particularly nasty cut or fracture as the result of a fall can cause direct infection of bone.

Once osteomyelitis develops, it is very difficult to cure. Many individuals develop a condition known as chronic osteomyelitis in which low-grade infection of bone continues for years. Symptoms include local pain, tenderness and swelling with occasional pussy drainage and fever. This disease requires sophisticated medical care.

Infected bone is weaker than normal bone. Activity such as running may aggravate infection, and runners should certainly never run with acute or recent onset osteomyelitis. Running with chronic osteomylitis should be discussed with a physician.

BONE BRUISE

Runners frequently develop bone bruise of the heel bone. This injury is discussed in Chapter 5.

FRACTURED BONE

Complete bone fracture is a relatively rare runners' injury. When it does occur, the most commonly involved bones are the toes and those around the ankle joint. For further discussion see Chapters 5 and 6.

TENDONS

Basic Structure

Tendons are strong sinewy structures that connect muscles to bone. They are composed primarily of fibers of connective tissue (collagen) which provide elasticity and strength. In some areas of the body, tendons run through tunnels or sheaths that act as a lining to facilitate a smooth gliding movement. Blood supply to tendons is relatively poor, and for this reason some tendon injuries require a long time to heal.

Training Adaptations

Tendons gradually thicken and become stronger with added stress of exercise. This is a relatively slow process which may require several months.

Tendon Injuries

Most tendon injuries are the result of overuse or poor conditioning. Adequate warm-up and stretching exercises are good preventive measures. The main tendon injury of concern to runners is tendinitis.

TENDINITIS

Cause: Tendinitis means inflammation of a tendon. Excessive stress on tendons from high mileage running causes minor degrees of damage resulting in inflammation of these structures. This common overuse injury plagues runners, especially beginners, whose tendons have not become strong enough to withstand the increased stresses of long distance running. In addition, direct pressure or irritation of a tendon can produce inflammation between the tendon and its sheath. Running shoes can cause tendinitis of the tendons on the top of the foot or the Achilles tendon of the heel. These and the tendons around the knee joint are the most common sites for runners' tendinitis (see Chapters 5 and 8 for further discussion).

Symptoms and Diagnosis: Pain, tenderness and swelling are usually well localized to the area of inflamed tendon. Pain often subsides after initial warm-up exercise, only to return with greater vengeance after a runner cools down.

Tendinitis must be differentiated from injuries such as sprains and joint inflammation. Although tendinitis symptoms are generally more discreetly localized than these other injuries, this diagnosis sometimes requires the expert knowledge of a physician who can pinpoint the problem.

Comments and Treatment: Rest, apply ice packs, and take aspirin to decrease the inflammation. Continue this regimen for 2 days following the development of tendinitis. If the symptoms improve, resume running. In fact, many mild cases of tendinitis will improve slowly without a break in training. In these instances, apply ice to the tender area immediately after each workout to limit the local inflammation. An adequate warm-up and stretching period is particularly important to prevent as well as to treat the inflammation.

Runners with chronic tendinitis frequently note improvement in their symptoms when hot packs are placed on the inflamed tendon for 15 minutes prior to a workout. Be certain that running shoes are not producing local irritation of an inflamed tendon.

TENDON TEAR AND COMPLETE RUPTURE

A tear or complete rupture of a tendon are relatively unusual runners' injuries. These problems usually arise in conjunction with a compound injury such as a fractured ankle. Severe tendon injuries produce pain and inability to use the involved muscle and usually require expert medical care by an orthopedic surgeon.

LIGAMENTS

Basic Structure

Ligaments are supporting structures around joints which help maintain stability. They are composed primarily of collagen and have limited elasticity.

Training Adaptations

During training, ligaments, like tendons, slowly become stronger and more able to handle the stresses of running.

Ligament Injuries

The main injuries of ligaments are: stretch, sprain or tear of the ligament.

SPRAINED LIGAMENTS

Cause: Ligaments are sprained when they are stretched beyond their normal range of motion. This injury usually occurs when a runner trips or stumbles, causing sudden twisting of a joint. The ankle and the knee joints are the most frequent sites of runners' sprains. The severity of a sprain injury varies considerably from mild pain to complete disability.

Symptoms and Diagnosis: Much of the disability is due to damage of surrounding blood vessels. Bleeding and local fluid accumulation in the tissues cause swelling and pain.

Runners who develop a severe sprain following a fall are often unable to bear weight because of instability of their ankle or knee joints and are therefore unable to walk, much less continue running. Less severe injuries may cause only minor incapacitation at the time of initial injury. Soon, however, bleeding and tissue swelling produce pain and disability.

Sprains around joints must be differentiated from more severe injuries such as fractures. Following the initial treatment of ligament sprains, more complete evaluation including X rays may be necessary.

Comments and Treatment: Immediate treatment to minimize bleeding and local swelling will decrease the degree of disability and speed recovery. Never try to run or walk off this injury, regardless of your stoical capacity to tolerate pain. Wrap the injured joint with an elastic bandage and cool it with an ice pack. Elevate the leg above the level of the hips. In addition, immobilize the leg with a blanket, pillow or splint until thorough medical evaluation is available. (See Chapters 6 and 8 for further discussion.)

TORN LIGAMENTS

Severe trauma may irreversibly stretch or tear a ligament. Runners most commonly tear ligaments in the ankle region following a severe sprain, and in the knee after an old injury of that joint. (For further discussion see Chapters 6 and 8.)

JOINTS

Basic Structure

Joints are structures which connect the ends of two or more bones to allow body motion. Within a joint space, the ends of the bones are covered by cartilage, a smooth slippery substance that constantly regenerates itself so that areas worn down by activity can be replaced.

The joint is surrounded by a thin membrane called synovial tissue that secretes lubricating fluid (synovial fluid) into the joint space, which minimizes friction associated with motion and also supplies nourishment to cartilage. In addition, the synovial tissue functions as a filter to remove small pieces of cartilage, blood and germs which may enter the joint.

Outside the synovial lining is a thick fibrous structure called the joint capsule which is connected to the ends of the bones and, together with ligaments surrounding the joint, helps give stability to the joint.

Joint Injuries

Runners frequently develop injuries to the hip, knee and ankle joints as well as to many of the small joints of the feet. The main joint problems to be considered are: synovitis (inflammation of the synovium), capsulitis (inflammation of the capsule), degenerative arthritis (damage of the cartilage within the joint) and dislocation of the joint.

SYNOVITIS (INFLAMMATION OF THE SYNOVIUM)

Cause: The synovial tissue is extremely sensitive to changes that occur within a joint. Infection, injury, bruise, overuse of a joint and direct pressure will all cause inflammation and synovitis. The synovial membrane reacts to injury by producing excess joint fluid resulting in "water on the joint" as well as local pain and tenderness. Synovitis may be an acute process resulting from injury or overuse, or it may represent a chronic problem associated with underlying damage to the effected joint.

Symptoms and Diagnosis: Synovitis produces pain, tenderness and swelling of the involved joint. These symptoms are aggravated by running and partially relieved by rest. The pain is often described as a dull, constant ache involving the whole joint.

Because synovitis usually causes diffuse joint pain, it can be distinguished from bursitis, tendinitis or ligament problems which cause localized pain. The main diagnostic problem, therefore, is to pinpoint the underlying cause of a runner's synovitis.

Comments and Treatment: Rest, take aspirin, wrap the joint with a compression bandage and apply ice packs. More severe cases may require drainage of the joint space. Sometimes a physician will recommend cortisone taken orally or injected directly into the joint, and although this medication is sometimes extremely helpful, there are many dangerous side effects that limit its usefulness. Chronic or recurrent synovitis suggests internal disease of the joint, which should be treated by a specialist (orthopedic surgeon or rheumatologist).

For further discussion, see the specific sections describing synovitis of the ankle, knee and hip joints.

CAPSULITIS (INFLAMMATION OF THE CAPSULE OF A JOINT)

A sudden stretch, twist of the joint, or similar action can cause capsulitis. In contrast to the synovium, the blood supply to the capsule is relatively meager. Therefore, recovery from capsulitis requires a longer period of time.

Runners develop capsulitis most commonly in the hip joint (see Chapter 10).

ARTHRITIS

Cause: If a joint is injured so that the cartilage can no longer repair itself, the two opposing joint surfaces will become roughened. This loss of cartilage and irregularity of bone within a joint space is called degenerative arthritis, a condition present to some extent in everyone above the age of twenty. Some people, however, are more prone to the development of serious degenerative arthritis and resulting disability. Predisposing factors include obesity, abnormal stress on the joint, injury to the joint, and a developmental abnormality of the joint.

Arthritis of the joint space causes inflammation which, in turn, causes further cartilage damage and breakdown. This vicious cycle leads to further degeneration of cartilage. Irritation of the synovium results in fluid accumulation as well as pain and tenderness of the joint.

Mild cases of degenerative arthritis usually improve through running. But severe arthritis, particularly of the knee and hip joints, may only be aggravated by it. However, there is no truth to the myth that running actually causes degenerative arthritis. To the contrary, there is some evidence that runners who ran during their youth have a lower incidence of degenerative arthritis than the normal population.

Symptoms and Diagnosis: While serious degenerative arthritis often produces pain and local inflammation of the joint, mild cases usually cause no problems. A runner may note vague aches within an involved joint space, sometimes accompanied by swelling. Occasionally there is a history of trauma to that joint, particularly in a case of arthritis of the knee.

Degenerative arthritis must be differentiated from other causes of arthritis such as rheumatoid arthritis and gout. (See Chapter 20 for further discussion of the different types of arthritis.)

Comments and Treatments: Degenerative arthritis should be treated with rest and aspirin to control inflammation. Often, even runners with mild cases should consult a physician to determine whether the condition has an underlying cause that can be corrected and to plan a reasonable running program.

Some individuals have such severe arthritis of the knee or hip that they are unable to run at all and must choose another aerobic exercise such as swimming in order to maintain cardiovascular fitness.

(Also see the specific sections on degenerative arthritis of the knee and hip.)

JOINT DISLOCATION

When the two opposing ends of bone within a joint slip out of their normal anatomical alignment, the joint is dislocated and is usually not capable of normal movement. The patella bone in front of the knee is the only structure that runners commonly dislocate. (See Chapter 8 for further discussion.)

BURSA

Basic Structure

Joints are surrounded by special closed sacs called "bursa" which facilitate the movement of muscles, tendons and ligaments. These sacs are lined by synovial tissue similar to that found in joints, and in some instances the cavities communicate with the main joint space.

Bursa sacs can become inflamed from overuse or direct injury. Runners may develop this condition—which is called bursitis —in the heel, hip joint or knee. It causes local pain and swelling over the involved bursa. (For further discussion, see chapters dealing with the heel, knee and hip.)

FASCIA

The loose connective tissue that surrounds muscle and acts as a cushion between adjacent ligaments and tendons is called fascia. It may become inflamed, a condition known as fasciitis. Runners develop fasciitis of the plantar fascia beneath the skin on the sole of the foot. (See Chapter 5 for further discussion of this particularly disabling injury.)

5

The Foot

No part of the body is more vital to a runner than his feet. These marvelous extremities are slammed on the ground thousands of times every day, absorbing shock forces that would destroy the strongest man-made machinery. It is therefore not surprising that foot injuries are among the most common of runners' ailments.

Basic Structure

The foot is composed of twenty-eight bones held together by small ligaments. The seven large tarsal bones make up the back half of the foot, while the metatarsal bones which connect to the toes comprise the front of the foot (Figure 5-1). The bones are arranged so that there are two arches which bear most of the body's weight. The long or longitudinal arch runs from the heel to the end of the metatarsals, while the transverse or metatarsal arch runs across the tip of the metatarsal bones from the large to the small toe.

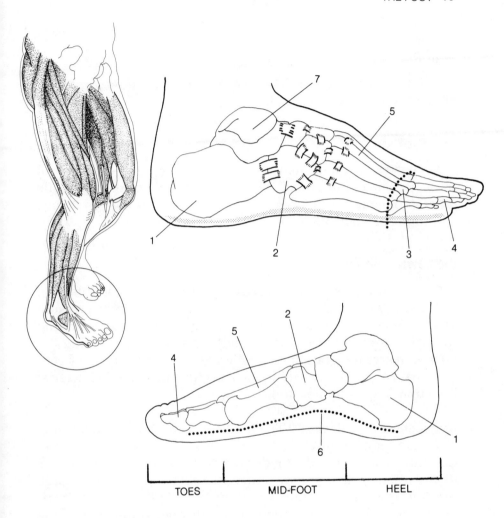

1 CALCANEUS BONE (HEEL)

2 TARSAL BONES

3 METATARSAL ARCH

4 TOES

5 METATARSAL BONES

6 LONGITUDINAL ARCH

7 TALUS

Figure 5-1.   THE FOOT

Foot Problems

Runner's foot problems can be divided into three broad regions: toe, mid-foot and heel.

Toe Problems

Many diseases and deformities can affect the toes. Some of these are due to individual variations in the shape of toes, while other problems result from the stresses of running, infections and improper care of toenails.

INGROWN TOENAIL

Cause: An ingrown toenail may result from chronic infection of the nail resulting in abnormal nail growth, or from pressure on the toes from tight shoes, in which case the skin surrounding the nail margin grows over the nail. The skin surrounding the area of overgrowth becomes swollen and inflamed, causing redness, pain and drainage along the margin of the toenail. Bacterial infection frequently develops.

Symptoms and Diagnosis: The large toe is the most common site. The pain may be so severe that the individual is unable to run. Careful examination of a tender toe will reveal that the margins of the toenail have grown under the skin. A pussy discharge usually indicates infection which, if there is fever, can be serious. Occasionally, X ray diagnosis will reveal infection of the bone underlying the nail.

Comments and Treatment: Prevention of ingrown toenails is an important part of a runner's routine personal hygiene. Toenails should be cut frequently. The edge should be trimmed in a straight line rather than along the natural curve of the toe (Figure 5-2). The toe box of a running shoe should be wide enough to prevent chronic pressure on the toenail.

If toenails are ingrown, soak them in warm water for 15 minutes at least three times a day. Then place a small wedge of

CUTTING TOENAILS Cut toenails straight across, not along contour of toe.

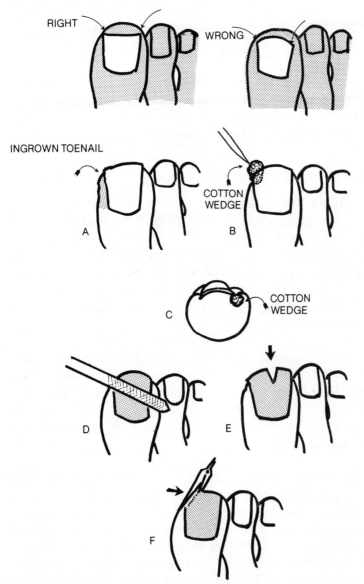

INGROWN TOENAIL: A. Site of redness and tenderness. B and C. Piece of cotton wedged under nail to relieve pressure. D. Thick, rough nail should be filed. E. Wedge cut in middle of nail will relieve pressure. F. Trim edge of ingrown nail.

Figure 5-2. TOENAILS

cotton between the nail and skin to correct the nail's growth (Figure 5-2). File the involved margin of the nail if it has thickened, and trim irregular edges. You may temporarily relieve the pressure by cutting a wedge in the middle of the nail (Figure 5-2).

More chronic cases require medical attention. Infection must be treated with antibiotics. Partial surgical removal of an ingrown toenail is sometimes necessary for severe cases, and this surgery usually brings dramatic relief.

BLACK TOENAILS (SUBUNGUAL HEMATOMA)

Cause: Runners frequently develop bleeding under a toenail from chronic friction, rubbing or bumping of the nail against the end of improperly fitting shoes. This condition may develop suddenly during a race or a long run, or it may be the result of chronic irritation which produced a blister that slowly extended from the tip to the underside of the nail. Other cases occur when the toe is stubbed against a hard object, causing a blood clot under the toenail.

Symptoms and Diagnosis: In some instances, when the condition has developed slowly over a period of time, there is no pain or discomfort. In most cases, however, pressure in the space under the toenail causes exquisite pain and tenderness. The painful toenail turns partially or completely black or red, and the toe will throb.

Comments and Treatment: This extremely uncomfortable condition is often avoidable. Be certain that shoes fit properly, with toe boxes of adequate width and height. Calluses or blisters on the tip of a toe are clues that there is chronic friction in that area during running, possibly caused by poorly fitted shoes. If necessary, protect toenails with felt pads or thick socks, but be careful because socks may wrinkle occasionally and cause friction at the tip of the toenail, leading to a blister in this area.

Once a blood clot has formed beneath a nail, the pressure must be relieved in order to alleviate the pain. First, carefully wash with soap and water and scrub the nail with tincture of iodine and 70% alcohol. Sterilize a sharp needle or paper clip by heating it in a flame until it is red hot, and use it immediately to melt the nail directly over the blood clot. As soon as the nail is punctured, the blood should escape with a sudden spurt as the pressure is mercifully relieved. Then soak the foot in warm water containing an antibacterial solution such as pHisoHex or Betadine. Once the foot is carefully dried, swab the hole with tincture of iodine and cover it with a sterile Band-Aid. Inspect it each day to make sure there is no infection.

A black toenail usually falls off. This may take several weeks to occur. The exposed nail bed is quite sensitive and should be protected until the nail has grown back. Therefore, never remove the old dead nail. If necessary, carefully tape it in place to assure its stability and protect the underlying tissue.

TOENAIL INFECTIONS

Fungal and bacterial infections of toenails are discussed in Chapter 13.

SPRAINED TOES

Cause: Toe sprains may result from stubbing the foot, stepping in a hole or banging the toes on a hard running surface. Sprains of the large toe frequently result from improper running form. Duck-footed runners place extra stress on the big toe as they push off, causing inflammation of the joint between the first metatarsal and the large toe.

Symptoms and Diagnosis: A runner with a sprained toe will note swelling and pain at the base of the toe. Running aggravates this symptom. Sometimes a runner will remember stubbing his toe. In other instances, sprains will develop during periods of increased mileage or following long runs on hard surfaces. Sprains occasionally have to be distinguished from broken toes and stress fractures of the metatarsals by X ray.

Comments and Treatment: Rest and apply ice to the injury for a few days. When the local inflammation subsides, running can be resumed. Treat sprains of the large toe with a toe spacer between the first and second toes (Figure 5-3), or tape in a "figure 8" to hold the toe out in a normal position. Half-inch paper tape will cause less skin irritation than adhesive tape. Treat sprains of the other toes with strapping. Tape these digits to a neighboring toe (Figure 5-3) with a wad of cotton placed between the toes to prevent local irritation.

BROKEN TOES

Cause: Runners occasionally break toes while running barefooted or by stepping on a rock or in a pothole. Most commonly, the small toe is broken while walking barefoot, catching it against some object and bending it sideways.

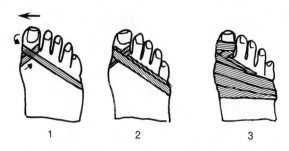

Large Toe Taping 1. Use ½-inch tape applied so that toe is pulled out to its normal position. 2. Repeat an overlapping figure-8 pattern with tape. 3. Complete the taping with strips tied around the foot.

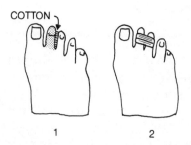

Minor Toe Taping 1. Place cotton between toes before taping. 2. Tape toe to neighbor for immobilization and support.

Figure 5-3. TAPING INJURED TOES

Symptoms and Diagnosis: Broken toes usually cause severe pain and swelling. There may also be bleeding into the soft tissue and a crunching sensation. A runner is usually actuely aware of the injury leading to the fracture. If you bend a toe in an unusual direction, fracture is likely. X rays should be obtained to confirm this diagnosis and to evaluate the extent of damage.

Comments and Treatment: Fractured toes usually require no specific treatment other than relief of pain. Running is often so painful that it is impossible for several days. Tape a fractured toe to an adjacent one just as you would for a sprained toe. A shoe with a rigid sole such as a construction boot often provides enough relief to enable walking and short distance running. But if pain becomes a major problem, a cast is sometimes advisable to immobilize the foot and allow adequate healing.

Pain is the main indicator of when to resume walking and jogging safely. If there is little discomfort, go ahead and run.

BUNIONS

Cause: The shift of the large toe toward the middle of the foot causes a deformity known as a bunion. Some individuals have an inherited tendency toward bunions, while others develop this problem from wearing tight shoes. When the large toe deviates to the center of the foot, the head of the first metatarsal bone becomes quite prominent along the inside of the foot (Figure 5-4). This bony prominence becomes irritated when it rubs against the shoe during running and walking. A bunion can result in degenerative arthritis of the joint of the great toe. Severe cases can also interfere with normal walking and running because the normal push-off motion of the great toe is lost.

Symptoms and Diagnosis: Most bunions result in pain, tenderness and swelling over the head of the first metatarsal bone, as well as irritation of the skin overlying this bone. The appearance of a bunion of the large toe is quite characteristic. The large toe is displaced toward the middle of the foot, and the first metatar-

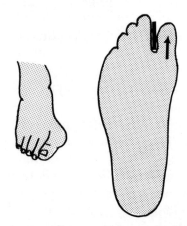

Large Toe Bunion A toe spacer of sponge rubber will help straighten the toe. Start with small spacer, then gradually widen it until toe is straight.

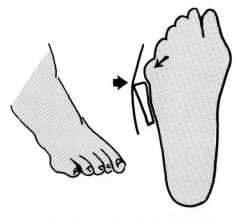

Tailor Bunion Protect bunion with a piece of adhesive felt 2 inches x ½ inch, applied directly behind bunion to relieve pressure from shoe.

Figure 5-4. BUNION AIDS

sal head is quite prominent (Figure 5-4). X rays may be necessary to define the degree of deformity.

Comments and Treatment: Mild bunions can be treated adequately by the use of proper footwear. The toe box should be wide enough to prevent compression of the toes. A toe spacer or bunion pad between the first and second toes is an effective device to shift the big toe back to its normal position (Figure 5-4). If a first metatarsal joint has become tender and inflamed, use a donut pad to relieve painful irritation.

Severe disabling bunions require surgical reconstruction of bones and ligaments resulting in a 2–4 month period of immobilization and decreased activity. Before surgery, a runner should thoroughly discuss the expectations and benefits of this treatment with his doctor.

TAILOR'S BUNION (BUNIONETTE)

Cause: Tailor's bunion is an enlargement of the base or end of the fifth metatarsal head, similar to that found in the previously described bunion of the first metatarsal (Figure 5-4). The name traces its origin to the days before sewing machines when tailors would sit cross-legged while they worked, causing friction over this bone and the gradual development of swelling and tenderness. Chronic friction from tight shoes may cause tailor's bunion in runners. Occasionally, prominence of this bone is due to a congenital enlargement.

Symptoms and Diagnosis: Pain, swelling and tenderness on the side of the foot directly over the fifth metatarsal indicate a tailor's bunion. A corn or callus is sometimes also present in this area. On occasion, X rays are required to define whether the source of irritation is from the soft tissue or from bony enlargement.

Comments and Treatment: This deformity is usually most effectively treated by obtaining shoes of adequate width to prevent pressure over the involved bone. Donut pads help protect the sensitive area, especially if a corn has developed. In more severe deformity, surgical correction may be indicated.

HAMMERTOE

A deformity of a single toe resulting in a hammerlike shape is referred to as a hammertoe. It may be inherited, or it may be the result of chronic compression of a toe from a short shoe.

This deformity is usually painfree. If there is discomfort, a corn or callus has probably developed directly over the middle joint of the involved toe. Runners who have a hammertoe should be sure that the toe box of their running shoes is adequate enough to prevent friction which would cause a corn on the skin overlying a deformed toe.

Claw toes refer to the development of hammertoe deformities in all of the toes of the foot.

MORTON'S SYNDROME

This so-called abnormality is perhaps one of the most misunderstood and overrated of all of a runner's problems. Morton hypothesized that a short first metatarsal bone caused pain and tenderness over the second and third metatarsals with associated callus formation. The problem was further thought to cause "weak feet" with instability and poor function of the arches. The validity of this observation has been disputed for years. Since approximately 80 percent of human feet have the so-called abnormally short first metatarsal bone, it seems absurd to define the condition as an abnormality. Moreover, many chronic foot problems that defy routine analysis have been wrongly attributed to Morton's foot. This appears to be an easy way out of a more scientific approach to runners' foot problems.

Mid-Foot Problems

FOOT SPRAIN

Cause: Runners frequently develop sprains of the foot. These injuries may result from high mileage, running on hard surfaces or sudden twisting or turning of the foot on irregular terrain. Any one of the small ligaments that interconnect the tarsal bones may be injured (Figure 5-1). Sprains of the metatarsal arch are the most common of runners' sprains, and these most often occur early in the season when runners begin to increase their mileage. Runners who develop sprains of the long arch may have some pre-existing deformity of this arch. A sprain of the plantar fascia, the strong connective tissue running along the bottom of the foot, may cause chronic plantar fasciitis (see below).

Symptoms and Diagnosis: A sprain causes pain over the injured ligament. Swelling and mild redness may also be present. Sprains of the long arch cause pain on the inside of the foot when you put weight on it. Movement of the injured joint increases the pain. Sprains must be distinguished from stress fractures and from tendinitis. While X rays help exclude stress fractures, it is often difficult to differentiate sprains from chronic tendinitis.

Comments and Treatment: Minor sprains usually respond quickly to decreased activity. More severe cases are best treated with pads, orthotics or arch supports to support the injured area until healing has occurred. Very severe cases require abstinence from running.

For a sprain of the metatarsal arch, place adhesive tape around the foot over the metatarsal heads in a circular manner, allowing for adequate spread of the foot during weight bearing. Metatarsal pads are also helpful (Figure 5-5). Sprains of the long arch usually respond to orthotics or arch supports. In addition, exercises to strengthen the arches are helpful. Perform them in stocking feet, preferably on a carpet.

1. Exaggerate pigeon-toe walking; that is, walk with toes turned in, actually placing one foot across the other. Walk 10 yards.

2. Walk 10 yards in a straight line, placing weight on the outer border of the feet.

3. Sit on chair and roll up a towel with your toes. Perform until muscles tire.

4. Pick up marbles or a pencil with your toes. Perform until muscles tire.

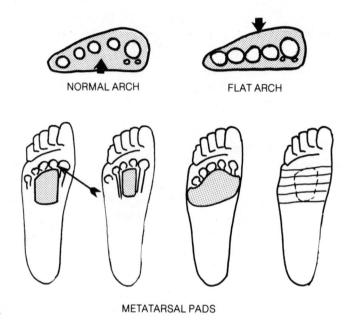

NORMAL ARCH   FLAT ARCH

METATARSAL PADS

A flat arch causes stress and pain on the head (end) of metatarsal bones. Cut adhesive felt pads to shape of foot and place directly behind (not over) the tender
metatarsal heads. Secure pads with adhesive tape.

Figure 5-5.   THE METATARSAL ARCH

PLANTAR FASCIITIS

Cause: Inflammation or small tears of the thick fascia connective tissue which runs along the bottom of the foot is called
plantar fasciitis (Figure 5-6). While the exact cause of this painful inflammation is unknown, it may become progressively incapacitating, resulting in the degeneration of the plantar fascia
and the growth of bony spurs in the area of the heel. This disease
is a common runners' lament that may result in prolonged disability.

Symptoms and Diagnosis: Pain and local tenderness usually develop on the sole near the heel, although they may occur any-
where from the heel to the metatarsals. There is frequently a

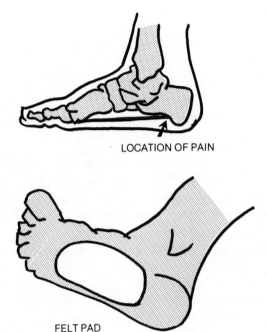

LOCATION OF PAIN

FELT PAD

Pain occurs in front part of heel, not where heel strikes ground. Felt pad or arch support lessens strain of fascia.

Figure 5-6. PLANTAR FASCIITIS

lump or swelling at the tender area. Plantar fasciitis must be differentiated from a bone spur, although these conditions frequently occur together, and from heel bruise.

Comments and Treatment: Plantar fasciitis is an overuse syndrome that develops slowly and may take many weeks to clear up. Since it frequently results from running on a hard surface or because of improper cushioning in the shoes, pay particular attention to these matters. If plantar fasciitis does occur, limit workouts to soft surfaces. Arch supports or felt pads will also help cushion the foot (Figure 5-6). Before a workout, soak the foot in tepid water for 15–20 minutes. After running, apply an ice pack to the tender area for at least 20 minutes. By following this routine, you may be able to control the problem in its early stages and prevent it from worsening, leading ultimately to severe disability.

When none of the simple measures is effective, seek professional medical attention. Injections of cortisone directly into the area of tenderness can sometimes alleviate this problem.

PAIN IN THE FOREFOOT (METATARSALGIA)

Cause: Pain in the area of the metatarsal bones at the ball of the foot is called metatarsalgia and may be caused by collapse of the transverse metatarsal arch, stress fracture of the metatarsal bones, or irritation of the nerves between the metatarsal bones.

1. Collapse of the transverse arch can result from improper footwear or from an inherited arch weakness. As a consequence, excessive weight is borne by the head of the metatarsals and calluses on the sole of the foot (Figure 5-5).

2. Stress fractures of the metatarsal bones are a common runners' problem which most often results from the trauma of long mileage runs combined with improper foot cushioning and running on hard surfaces. The second, third and fourth metatarsals are the most common sites of stress fractures (Figure 5-7).

3. Irritation of the nerves between the metatarsal bones is called Morton's neuroma. The nerve grows thicker, probably as a result of irritation caused by the rubbing together of the bones during running. Authorities think that this problem occurs only between the third and fourth metatarsal bones.

Symptoms and Diagnosis: The main symptom of metatarsalgia is, of course, pain in the ball of the foot. There are individual types of discomfort associated with the different causes of metatarsalgia.

1. Metatarsalgia due to a collapsed transverse arch usually causes chronic pain in the ball of the foot associated with callus in that area, and can be pinpointed by close inspection of the foot.

2. Stress fractures usually cause gradual development of pain in the forefoot without a history of trauma. Local swelling and tenderness are frequently present. The pain improves when a

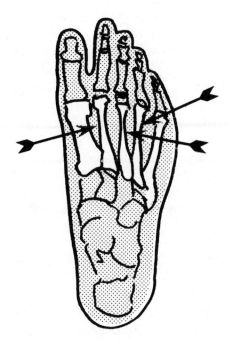

Most common sites of stress fracture of the foot are second, third, and fourth metatarsal bones.

Figure 5-7. METATARSAL STRESS FRACTURES

runner rests but returns when he resumes running. An X ray may or may not detect these hairline fractures.

3. Metatarsal nerve compression causes a unique burning, tingling or numbness between the third and fourth toes. These symptoms are usually relieved when walking barefoot or wearing loose-fitting shoes. Tight shoes aggravate the symptoms. A lump is often felt between the involved metatarsals, and this site is frequently tender. Squeezing the front of the foot together often produces the symptoms.

Comments and Treatment

1. Collapse of the metatarsal arch usually responds to a metatarsal arch support. You may have to try different types of pads until you find one that relieves the symptoms (Figure 5-5). These pads are usually cut from adhesive felt and then either taped to

the foot or placed into the shoe. They act as shock absorbers during weight bearing, taking the strain off the heads of the metatarsals, and should be worn until the symptoms completely disappear.

2. Stress fractures usually heal with no difficulty, making specific treatment often unnecessary. However, when severe pain continues a lightweight cast is sometimes necessary. Do not run for at least 3–4 weeks until the fracture has begun to heal.

3. Morton's neuroma usually improves when you wear shoes with a wider toe box. When the condition is more resistant to treatment, injection with cortisone may be beneficial, and severe cases may occasionally require surgical removal of the irritated nerve.

FLATFEET

Cause: Absence of the long arch of the feet is called "flatfeet" (Figure 5-8), a common condition that is frequently inherited. Running itself does not cause or lead to flatfeet.

Symptoms and Diagnosis: Runners with flatfeet may notice pain in the instep while running, although in many cases there are no symptoms. Moreover, many runners with flatfeet have an unusual running style or foot strike which may lead to pain in the foot, leg or knee. Examination of a runner's foot while he is standing will reveal a flatfoot. The central arch of the foot should clear the ground by at least one inch as it spans the weight-bearing areas of the metatarsals and the heel.

Comments and Treatment: Flatfeet require no specific therapy unless they are associated with pain, in which case orthotics and arch supports will usually provide adequate relief. A runner can fashion a homemade support from felt (Figure 5-8) or from orthoplast (Chapter 3).

TENDINITIS

Cause: The tendons on the top of the foot are frequently irritated and inflamed. This condition, known as tendinitis, usually

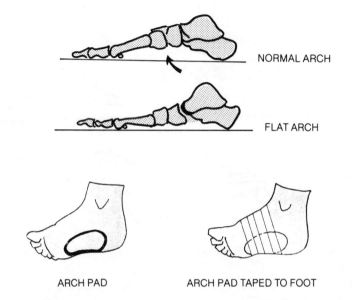

NORMAL ARCH

FLAT ARCH

ARCH PAD

ARCH PAD TAPED TO FOOT

A supporting arch pad should extend from the head of the first metatarsal to concavity of the heel. Tape should not be too tight.

Figure 5-8. FLATFOOT

results from tight shoes. Shoelaces may be tied too tightly, or the shoes themselves may be too narrow for the forefoot. Runners with high arches are particularly susceptible to this problem.

Symptoms and Diagnosis: Pain, irritation, swelling, local tenderness and a crunching sensation of the tendons along the top of the foot indicate tendinitis. Careful inspection of the tendons reveals that inflammation is responsible for a runner's discomfort.

Comments and Treatment: Tendinitis should disappear when the source of irritation is removed. Check shoes to make sure that the lacing is not digging into the tendons. Ladder-type lacing causes less irritation than the conventional cross lacing used by most runners. If a particular point of friction cannot be found in the running shoe, protect the tendons with felt pads or thicker

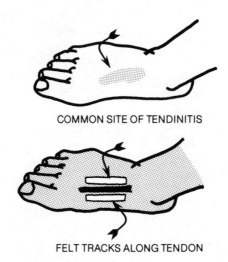

COMMON SITE OF TENDINITIS

FELT TRACKS ALONG TENDON

Place adhesive felt tracks ¼-inch thick x ½-inch wide on each side of swollen area to relieve pressure on tendon.

Figure 5-9. TENDINITIS ON TOP OF FOOT

running socks. Special felt strip "tracks" ¼-inch thick and ½-inch wide are easy to make and very effective (Figure 5-9). Place them on each side of the inflamed tendon to prevent pressure on the involved area. Wear them at all times, not just when running. In addition, aspirin will help relieve the inflammation. Apply ice packs to the inflamed area for at least 15 minutes after running.

Heel Problems

HEEL BRUISES

Cause: A runner can bruise his heel when he steps on a hard object such as a stone while running barefoot or while wearing thick running shoes. This injury can lead to bleeding in the tissues between the skin and the bone or bleeding in the periosteum tissue which covers the bone. Occasionally, a heel is bruised from running on a hard surface in thin-soled racing shoes.

Symptoms and Diagnosis: Heel bruises cause persistent pain and tenderness over the bottom of the heel following a relatively minor injury. This must be distinguished from plantar fasciitis, stress fracture of the heel bone (calcaneus), arthritis of one of the tarsal joints and inflammation of the insertion of the Achilles tendon. X rays (Figure 5-10) and careful examination by a physician are often required to exclude these other diseases.

Comments and Treatment: Mild heel bruises usually improve with adequate cushioning of the heel. More severe cases require a plastic heel cup to distribute the weight-bearing forces over a wider area. In addition, the heel can be supported with 1-inch wide, 8-inches long adhesive tape, used with or without a pad (Figure 5-11) and applied in an overlapping pattern for snug support.

To prevent heel bruises, never run long distances on hard surfaces in thin-soled shoes. Many brands of excellent, well-cushioned, lightweight long distance training and racing shoes are available.

BONE SPUR (CALCANEUS)

Cause: Bony growth extending from the heel bone (calcaneus) is common at the insertion of the plantar fascia as well as at the insertion of the Achilles tendon (Figure 5-10). These spurs usually cause no difficulty unless they are associated with plantar fasciitis.

Symptoms and Diagnosis: Bone spurs may cause pain and tenderness at the base of the calcaneus bone, particularly when deep pressure is applied to the sole of the foot. Very often runners with painful bone spurs have a history of chronic plantar fasciitis. In addition, X rays are helpful in making the diagnosis of bone spur. However, since there may be no symptoms and since bone spurs often result from chronic plantar fasciitis, positive X ray diagnosis does not always prove that the bone spur is responsible for the runner's symptoms.

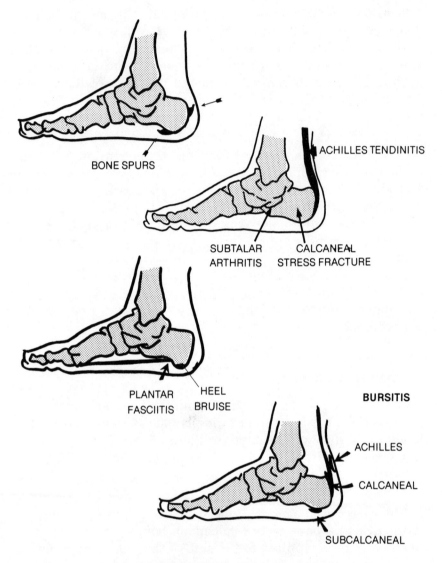

Heel pain can result from plantar fasciitis, heel bruise, heel bone spurs, subtalar arthritis, calcaneal stress fracture, Achilles tendinitis or bursitis.

Figure 5-10.   HEEL PROBLEMS

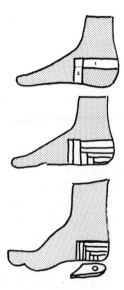

Bruised Heel Taping Using 1-inch tape, place first strip just below ankle and pull toward toes. Pull second strip up from under heel to overlap first. Cover heel with alternating, overlapping strips for snug support. May be used with heel pad.

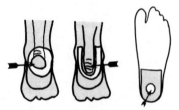

Felt Pads for Bursitis Place donut or U-shaped pads around inflamed bursa to eliminate pressure.

Heel Cup Plastic heel cups mold to the foot to relieve bursitis or bruise on bottom of heel.

Figure 5-11. TREATMENT OF HEEL PROBLEMS

Comments and Treatment: Heel bone spurs often respond to the padding methods described for heel bruise, plantar fasciitis and bursitis (see specific sections). In addition, arch supports help remove the pressure from the inflamed area. More resistant cases usually respond to cortisone injections, although a surgical repair occasionally may be necessary—a procedure requiring several months of complete rest.

BURSITIS OF THE HEEL

Cause: Bursitis of the heel can develop in the Achilles bursa, the calcaneus bursa or the subcalcaneus bursa (Figure 5-10). Inflammation of these bursa usually result from nonspecific irritation during running.

Symptoms and Diagnosis: Localized pain, swelling and tenderness are usually present over the involved area. Bursitis must be differentiated from bone spurs and tendinitis, and this distinction is frequently very difficult. However, the treatment programs for these conditions are quite similar.

Comments and Treatment: Bursitis usually responds to a combination of aspirin for anti-inflammatory action as well as icepack treatment after running. Removal of fluid from the inflamed bursa and injection of cortisone is often curative. A donut or U-shaped felt pad surrounding the bursa will eliminate the pressure on this area and facilitate healing (Figure 5-11).

6

The Ankle

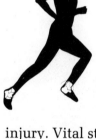

Runner's ankles are relatively vulnerable to injury. Vital structures such as tendons, blood vessels and nerves are close to the surface of the skin and, therefore, more prone to injury than they are in the leg where they are covered by a protective layer of muscles. Ankle injuries can completely disable the best of runners and often take several months to heal.

Basic Structure

Functionally speaking, it is best to consider the true ankle joint together with the talo-calcaneal joint which lies just below it (Figure 6-1). The ends of the tibia and fibula leg bones form an arch surrounding the top of the talus bone. This ankle joint can move in only one direction, flexing or extending the foot up or down. Side-to-side motion of the foot normally occurs in the talo-calcaneal joint. Some lateral movement is essential for proper running technique. Surrounding these bones are powerful ligaments: the lateral collateral ligaments on the outside of the foot and the deltoid ligaments on the inside. A thick capsule of connective tissue provides stability in the front and back of the ankle.

95

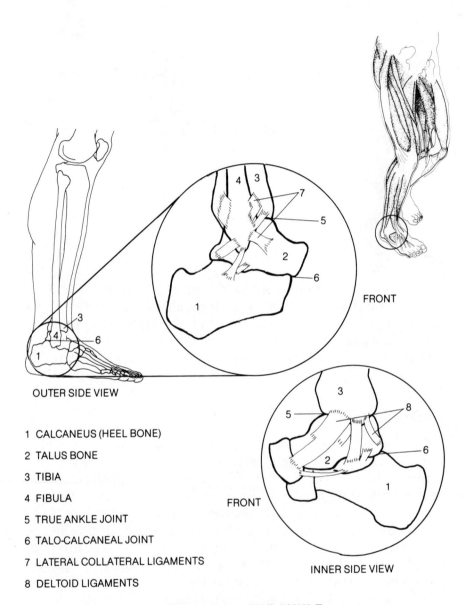

OUTER SIDE VIEW

FRONT

FRONT

INNER SIDE VIEW

1 CALCANEUS (HEEL BONE)

2 TALUS BONE

3 TIBIA

4 FIBULA

5 TRUE ANKLE JOINT

6 TALO-CALCANEAL JOINT

7 LATERAL COLLATERAL LIGAMENTS

8 DELTOID LIGAMENTS

Figure 6-1.   THE ANKLE

Injuries of the Ankle

ANKLE CONTUSION AND LOCAL HEMATOMA

Cause: Since blood vessels in the area of the ankle are close to the skin, a local blow or contusion can rupture a small vein or artery, producing local bleeding under the skin (hematoma).

Symptoms and Diagnosis: Pain and dramatic local swelling develop rapidly after a mild sprain or local blow to the ankle joint. The site of swelling may be above, below or directly at the ankle joint.

Comments and Treatment: Immediately try to minimize the degree of swelling by elevating the leg, wrapping the ankle with a firm compressive bandage, and applying an ice pack (Figure 6-2) for at least 2 hours, allowing 5–10 minutes rest period every half hour to avoid frostbite. Often the initial dramatic swelling will almost disappear following the prompt application of a compressive wrap and ice. A local bruise or blue spot will usually remain for a few days after the initial injury. A local hematoma can usually be distinguished from more serious ankle injuries by the fact that there is only minor pain and discomfort associated with this injury. It is usually safe to resume running the day after the injury. If a runner does not treat an ankle contusion promptly, the swelling can lead to several days of disability.

ANKLE SPRAIN

Cause: An injury that stretches or tears the ligaments surrounding the ankle is called a sprain. While this can occur on either the inner or outer side of the ankle, when there is forceful twisting of the foot, most ankle sprains do occur on the outside of the joint. Runners often develop this injury from stepping in a hole or on an irregular object. The resulting ligamentous injury may vary from a mild stretch to a tear or complete rupture. Ankle sprains are usually classified as: type 1, a mild stretch; type 2, a

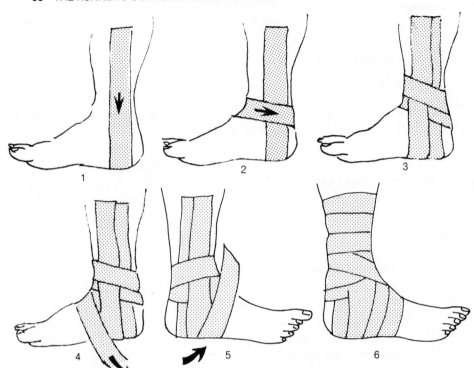

Ankle Taping (Inner side view 1-4; outer side view 5-6.) 1. Starting on inner side 6 inches above ankle, pull tape under heel to finish 6 inches above outer side. 2. Pull horizontal strip from top of foot around ankle. 3. Repeat with two or three more overlapping strips. 4. Start figure 8 on top inner side. 5. Pull under foot and anchor on ankle. Repeat figure 8's for support. 6. Apply anchor strips above and below ankle.

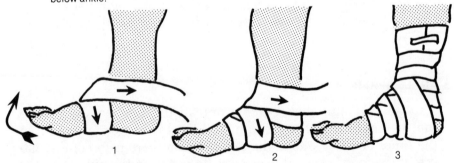

Ankle Compression Wrap 1. Stand with front of foot on edge of chair. Use 2- or 3-inch elastic bandage in a figure-8 wrap starting on inner side of foot. 2. Overlap repeated figure 8's for flat, snug wrap. 3. Complete wrap 8 inches above ankle. Secure with clips or tape. Do not apply too tightly.

Figure 6-2. ANKLE INJURIES

partial tear of the ligament; type 3, a complete tear of the ligament with instability of the ankle joint.

Symptoms and Diagnosis: An ankle sprain causes immediate pain after a runner stumbles, falls or trips while running over rough ground or after stepping in a hole. The initial pain may be mild, increasing during the next hour as local swelling develops. Swelling, local bleeding and a crunching sensation of the soft tissue over the ankle are common. With a severe type 3 sprain, the ankle also may be unstable. A sprain must be distinguished from a simple hematoma and a serious fracture of the ankle. Most severe cases require expert examination by a physician as well as X ray evaluation.

Comments and Treatment: Immediately stop running when you injure an ankle. Pain may not develop for several minutes after a relatively severe sprain, and the ankle can be further damaged by attempting to "run out" the injury. Initial treatment is the same as that prescribed for ankle contusion: stop running, elevate the leg, apply a compression wrap and an ice pack. This treatment is usually sufficient for a mild type 1 sprain. When pain and swelling persist, evaluation must be made by a physician.

Type 2 sprains should also be treated with a compression wrap or ankle taping (Figure 6-2) and application of ice for 48 hours, after which massage is often useful. Runners who are unable to bear weight on the injured ankle should use crutches for the first few days. Once pain and swelling have diminished, tape the ankle and begin to walk. Retape it daily. When weight bearing and walking are comfortable, jogging can be slowly resumed. Start gradually by jogging 25 yards, then walking 25 yards, and increasing the distance as tolerated. Treatment of type 2 ankle sprain may require 2–3 weeks of wrapping, icing and slow resumption of running. Before attempting to race, practice running tight figure-8 loops. This exercise stretches both the inside and outside of the ankles, helping to restore normal flexibility. Skipping rope is also an excellent aid to recovery.

The severe type 3 sprains usually require complete immobilization of the ankle with a cast. Healing of the injured ligaments requires 4–6 weeks, resulting in considerable muscle atrophy and weakness. Once the ankle sprain has healed, therefore, rehabilitation must include strengthening exercises for all of the muscles of the leg (see Chapter 3).

Some runners develop recurrent or chronic sprains of the ankle because of improper foot plant. They tend to land too far on the outside of the foot (Figure 6-3). A felt or rubber wedge along the outer border of the shoe will help to correct this problem. Other runners develop recurrent ankle sprains associated with chronic ankle instability (see section later in chapter).

ANKLE FRACTURE

Cause: Runners develop ankle fracture in much the same way that they develop sprains: by sudden twisting or turning of the foot while running. The fibula leg bone on the outside of the ankle is the most common site of this type of fracture. Fractures vary greatly in their severity—from small bone chips, which are usually no more difficult to treat than sprains, to severe fractures of several bones, which require surgical correction and many months to heal. Many fractures are associated with injuries to the tendons.

Symptoms and Diagnosis: A runner is quite aware of the injury that causes an ankle fracture. The two most common causes are tripping over a rock and falling into a pothole. Immediate severe pain develops with swelling and loss of normal ankle symmetry. The ankle is quite tender and a crunching sensation is felt at the site of the injury. A runner is usually unable to walk on a fractured ankle. A fractured ankle must be distinguished from a severe sprain. Examination by a physician and an X ray are required.

Comments and Treatment: The immediate treatment of a fractured ankle is immobilization. Wrap a pillow or blanket snugly around the ankle to provide support. Do not attempt to put weight on the injured ankle. To minimize local bleeding and swelling, elevate the leg and apply an ice pack.

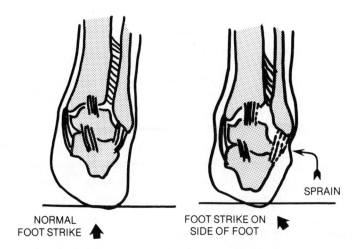

Abnormal rotation of the foot can stretch ligaments, causing sprain.

NORMAL
FOOT STRIKE

FOOT STRIKE ON
SIDE OF FOOT

SPRAIN

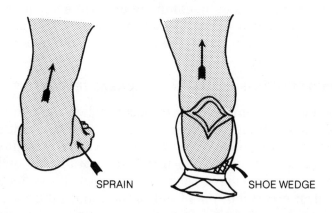

SPRAIN

SHOE WEDGE

Shoe wedge of felt or rubber will straighten ankle to prevent inward rotation.

Figure 6-3. ANKLE SPRAIN

Definitive treatment of a fractured ankle depends upon the severity of the injury. A cast may be adequate in some cases, while more severe damage may require surgical treatment with wires and screws to provide proper alignment of involved bones. It takes several months for an ankle fracture to heal. As with severe ankle sprains, muscle weakness will develop, and rehabilitation should include muscle-strengthening exercises.

TRICK ANKLE (CHRONIC INSTABILITY)

Cause: When old sprains are not allowed to heal adequately, loosening and stretching of the involved ligaments occur, producing an unstable ankle joint. The outer side of the ankle is the most common site of this problem.

Symptoms and Diagnosis: The ankle gives way or turns while you walk or run on rough ground. Runners with trick ankles often have a history of recurrent ankle sprains, with chronic swelling and tenderness over the outer side of their trick ankle.

Comments and Treatment: Sometimes you can obtain relief by taping the ankle or placing a lateral wedge in the shoe (Figure 6-3). If, however, this condition is severe enough that ankle instability continues, a more complete medical evaluation including X rays is necessary. These cases may require a surgical reconstructive procedure to strengthen the involved ligaments.

SNAPPING TENDON (SUBLUXATING PERONEAL TENDON)

This relatively unusual injury occurs when the peroneal tendons are dislocated from their normal groove behind the fibula component of the ankle (Figure 6-4). This usually results from a kick or blow, producing the initial dislocation. Following this injury, the tendon snaps back in place. But if no treatment is obtained, it may snap in and out of the groove during running. Painful tendon snapping is a chronic problem. Treatment requires either immobilization with a cast to maintain the tendon in the proper position during healing, or surgery to repair the damage.

TENDINITIS

Tendons that pass over the ankle may develop tendinitis from local irritation or injury, causing pain, swelling and tenderness. Treatment is similar to that outlined for tendinitis of tendons of the foot. Felt strip tracks help relieve the irritation and pressure on the tendon until healing occurs.

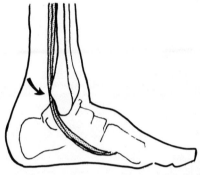

Normal location of tendon behind fibula

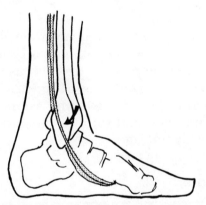

Subluxation of tendon over end of fibula

Figure 6-4.   PERONEAL TENDON SUBLUXATION

7

The Leg

Runners frequently develop leg injuries. Shin splints, stress fractures and pulled calf muscles are problems that sideline elite runners as well as casual joggers. Many of these injuries can be avoided by adherence to two basic training principles: perform daily stretching exercises to prevent tightening of leg muscles, and run on soft surfaces for a significant portion of weekly mileage.

Basic Structure

The leg joins the knee to the ankle joint (Figure 7-1) and is constructed of two leg bones: the tibia and the fibula, surrounded by several muscle groups that assist in the movement of the knee, ankle, and foot. The leg muscles are divided into four separate compartments by rigid sheaths of connective tissue— the anterior compartment, the lateral compartment on the side of the leg, the deep compartment and the superficial posterior compartment (Figure 7-2). Muscles in the superficial posterior compartment are the ones most frequently injured while running. (Figure 7-3). The soleus muscle runs from the top of the fibula and tibia to join the Achilles tendon which attaches to the heel and which flexes the foot downward. The plantaris, a small mus-

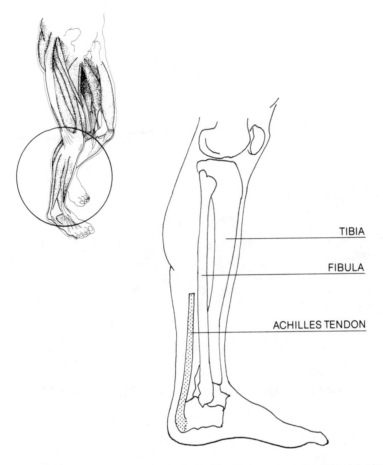

The tibia (shin) bone is the major leg bone. The fibula on the outer side of the leg is not weight bearing. The Achilles tendon connects the powerful calf muscles to the foot to enable push-off during running.

Figure 7-1. THE LEG

cle, runs from the back of the knee joint to form a long slender tendon going behind the major calf muscle to insert in the back of the heel. It flexes the foot downward and flexes the leg. The gastrocnemius is the main calf muscle. It arises as two heads from the bottom of the femur and forms the thick Achilles tendon (heel cord) which is the primary structure used for push-off during running.

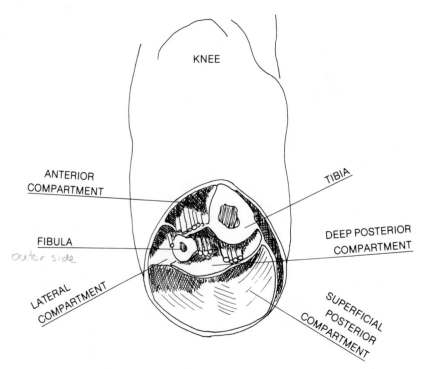

Figure 7-2. MUSCLE COMPARTMENTS OF THE LEG

Leg Problems

To aid the runner in self-diagnosis, injuries have been divided into calf problems and problems involving the bones and the front part of the leg.

Calf Problems

TIGHT CALF

Cause: The repetitive pushing-off action of running naturally tightens the calf muscles. When a runner does not gently stretch the muscles and tendons of his calf, they will become progressively tighter. Local soreness of the calf may develop. More im-

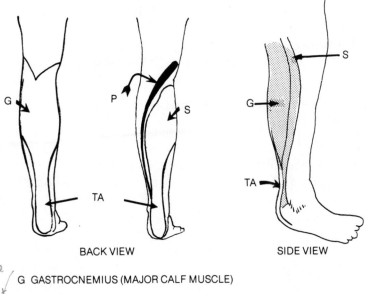

BACK VIEW   SIDE VIEW

G GASTROCNEMIUS (MAJOR CALF MUSCLE)

S SOLEUS

P PLANTARIS

TA ACHILLES TENDON

Superficial Posterior Compartment

Figure 7-3.   CALF MUSCLES

portant, tight calf muscles are susceptible to muscle pulls and tears, while tightness of the Achilles tendon can lead to tear or complete rupture of that vital structure.

Symptoms and Diagnosis: Beginning runners often develop tight calf muscles because they neglect a daily stretching program. Veteran runners can develop this problem when they increase their daily mileage or switch to hard running surfaces. Runners who have a high arch or who run high on their toes are more prone to tight calf muscles. Test the tightness of calf muscles by trying the heel cord stretch exercise described in Chapter 2. If there is pain and burning in the calf or Achilles tendon while performing this exercise, these structures are too tight.

Comments and Treatment: This condition is completely avoidable, but many runners are ignorant of the need to stretch calves and heel cords. A few minutes of stretching before and after running, or at any other time in the day, will prevent many painful injuries. Runners over the age of thirty are particularly susceptible to complications associated with tight heel cords.

CALF MUSCLE STRAIN (MUSCLE PULLS)

Cause: A strain or pulled muscle results from tearing of muscle fibers when they are stretched beyond their limits. Tight muscles are more susceptible to this injury. In addition to muscle injury, there may be damage to blood vessels resulting in local bleeding and swelling. The gastrocnemius, the soleus and the plantaris are the most common leg muscles pulled by runners.

Symptoms and Diagnosis: Runners most frequently pull calf muscles during speed work or races. They will feel a sudden pain in the calf, varying from a relatively mild discomfort to a sudden pop and burning sensation in the leg. The severity of the pain usually reflects the degree of the injury. There is also swelling and tightness of the calf muscles with local tenderness over the area of the injury.

A plantaris pull is most often felt in the upper middle portion of the calf, while a pull of the gastrocnemius may be felt at any place in the major calf muscle. A soleus pull is felt along the side of the calf between the shin bone and the major calf muscle.

Pulled calf muscles are easily diagnosed on the basis of the circumstances of the injury. Severe pulls must occasionally be differentiated from posterior compartment syndrome (described later) and complete rupture of the muscle or the Achilles tendon.

Comments and Treatment: Treat pulled muscles with compression, elevation and ice packs to minimize the degree of swelling and inflammation. After 48 hours, apply local heat, and if the pain has subsided, gradually resume your running program.

When a muscle pull occurs close to the attachment of the Achilles tendon, it is likely that the runner is running too high on his toes and that calf muscles are probably tight. A half-inch sponge heel inside the shoe will help lessen the tension on this group of muscles and temporarily relieve the pain. After a few days, begin stretching exercises to avoid recurrent injury.

ACHILLES TENDINITIS

Cause: The Achilles tendon may become inflamed from overuse, from running over unusual surfaces such as steep hills, or by increasing the weekly mileage too rapidly. Local irritation from running shoes can occasionally produce Achilles tendinitis. It is also a frequent injury in sports that require jumping such as basketball. Once again, tightness of the calf makes injury more likely.

Symptoms and Diagnosis: Pain develops over the Achilles tendon at the back of the heel (Figure 7-4), and there is usually tenderness and swelling as well. When the ankle is flexed and extended, a grating sensation may be felt, indicating friction between the tendon and its surrounding sheath.

Comments and Treatment: Runners who develop Achilles tendinitis should begin the usual therapy for tendinitis: take oral anti-inflammatory drugs such as aspirin, apply ice packs, and rest until acute inflammation has subsided. Mild cases may disappear when daily mileage is reduced. A ¾-inch heel lift helps decrease the stretch of the tendon, thereby minimizing inflammation. Once the pain has disappeared, start a gradual stretching program.

Be certain to select running shoes that possess good shock-absorbing characteristics. Also, examine them carefully to make

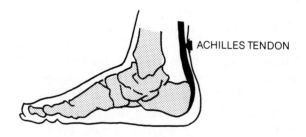

ACHILLES TENDON

Pain may occur at any site along lower quarter of heel cord.

Figure 7-4. ACHILLES TENDINITIS

sure that there is no external pressure point which irritates the Achilles tendon.

RUPTURED ACHILLES TENDON

Runners over the age of thirty must be particularly conscientious about performing daily stretching exercises. As we age, our tendons lose some of their elastic properties. The Achilles tendon is particularly susceptible to complete rupture and this injury is common among older athletes. Therefore, gentle heel cord stretching is especially important before any run, particularly a race.

Rupture of the Achilles tendon causes sudden excruciating pain. In fact, stricken runners think they have been shot. Casting or surgical repair is necessary to treat this injury, requiring a recovery period of several months.

SUPERFICIAL POSTERIOR COMPARTMENT SYNDROME

A compartment syndrome that usually involves the deep posterior compartment (described later) occasionally afflicts the superficial posterior compartment of the leg. With the exception of the location, this injury is essentially the same as that described below.

Bone and Anterior Leg Injuries

SHIN SPLINTS

The term "shin splints" refers to pain that occurs along the lower third of the inner side of the tibia or shin bone (Figure 7-5). It is actually a vague term, describing only the location of the pain. Since the problem can result from a variety of injuries, a runner must pinpoint the cause of shin splints in order to alleviate and prevent recurrence. For this reason, think in terms of specific injuries rather than the vague terminology shin splints. There are three types of injuries that cause shin splints: stress fracture of the tibia, soft tissue inflammation (periostitis,

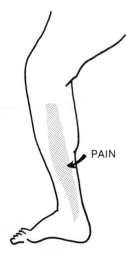

PAIN

Pain is localized in the lower third of the inner shin.

Figure 7-5.   SHIN SPLINTS

myositis and fasciitis) and deep posterior compartment syndrome. These different problems are outlined on Table 7-1.

STRESS FRACTURE OF THE TIBIA

Cause: A small break in the bony substance of the tibia bone is
an overuse injury. While these stress fractures can occur at any
location along the shaft of the tibia, they are found most frequently at the tend of the tibia near the ankle, the area where
shin splints occur. Runners develop tibial stress fractures from
running on hard surfaces and from high mileage running. Beginning runners suffer stress fractures when they don't allow
enough time for their bones to adapt to running. Rapidly increased mileage overstresses bone that has not had time to re-
organize and strengthen its internal structure (see Chapter 4).

Symptoms and Diagnosis: Runners note the gradual onset of
pain localized to the involved area of bone. Symptoms begin as

TABLE 7-1

Shin Splints

	Tibia Stress Fracture	Soft Tissue Inflammation—Periostitis, Myositis, Fasciitis	Deep Posterior Compartment Syndrome
CAUSE:	Overuse, high mileage, hard running surface	Overuse, high mileage, hard running surface, toe-out running style	Tight muscle compartment
RUNNING SYMPTOMS:	Pain with running, accentuated by downhill runs and deceleration; relieved with rest	Pain during running; relieved by overnight rest	Pain at end of run, accentuated by toe-off; continues at rest
LOCAL PAIN AND TENDERNESS:	Lower one-third tibia	Lower one-third tibia	Lower one-third tibia
DIAGNOSIS:	Local swelling common No muscle atrophy	Increased circumference of leg at pain level Muscle atrophy common	No swelling No muscle atrophy
X RAY:	Positive in 2–4 weeks	Negative	Negative
ISOTOPE BONE SCAN:	Positive	Negative	Negative

TREATMENT:	1. Rest—4–6 weeks
	   Casting
	2. Rehabilitation and muscle strengthening exercises
	3. Soft running surface
	   Well-cushioned shoes
		1. Reverse ankle wrap
		   Ice
		   Aspirin
		2. Change running form
		   Muscle strengthening exercises
		   Soft running surface
			Surgery (Fasciotomy)

a dull ache, gradually increasing in intensity. Typically, the pain will decrease at night only to return again during walking or running. Downhill running and deceleration are particularly painful.

There is usually a localized area of tenderness and mild swelling over the involved site. As with other stress fractures, X rays are usually not diagnostic during the early stages of this injury. Radioactive bone scans help detect this cause of shin splints (see Chapter 4).

Comments and Treatment: Stress fractures of the tibia occasionally progress to complete break of the bone. Since the tibia is one of the most important weight-bearing bones of the lower extremities, this injury should be carefully treated. The leg is often placed in a cast for several weeks until healing has occurred. Following recovery from injury, rehabilitation therapy must include exercises to strengthen the leg muscles. Runners who have sustained stress fractures of the tibia should gradually resume running, and they should try to run only on soft surfaces. Training sessions on hard surfaces should be slowly integrated into the program, allowing the bone time to adjust to this stress.

PERIOSTITIS, MYOSITIS, AND FASCIITIS

Cause: Periostitis, another possible cause of shin splints, represents inflammation of the tissue (periosteum) that surrounds bone. The most common site of periostitis is along the inner end of the tibial bone. Most authorities agree that this overuse injury is a precursor to stress fracture. Its causes are similar to those that produce tibial stress fracture. However, some cases of shin splints are thought to be caused by inflammation of the muscles of the deep posterior compartment of the leg (myositis) and by inflammation of the fascia surrounding this compartment (fasciitis). These injuries can be lumped together with periostitis as soft tissue inflammation shin splints.

Symptoms and Diagnosis: Diffuse pain, tenderness and swelling are usually located over the lower third of the inner margin of the shin bone. Often both legs are affected. Pain increases during running and is relieved during rest. Atrophy of muscle is sometimes present. This condition may become chronic, leading to increasingly severe discomfort.

Comments and Treatment: Treat periostitis early before a chronic injury develops. A reverse ankle wrap (Figure 7-6), local ice packs and anti-inflammatory medications such as aspirin, will give initial relief of symptoms. Severe cases are treated by restriction of running until pain disappears. Runners should pay particular attention to their running styles. Duck-footed gait must be corrected. Orthotics are often used to adjust the foot and heel strike, reducing the stress on the involved area.

Experienced runners sometimes develop periostitis when they change from one type of running surface to another. Indoor tracks with hard surfaces and tight curves are particularly hazardous. The additional stress placed on the inside or left leg often causes shin splints of this extremity. Turtle-backed roads produce pain in the right or left leg as described in Chapter 2, Figure 2-3. Understanding these problems will enable a runner to alternate his regimen to prevent new stresses from causing injury. Any runner who develops shin splints should try to run on grass and soft running surfaces as frequently as possible and wear only well-cushioned running shoes.

DEEP POSTERIOR COMPARTMENT SYNDROME

Cause: The muscles of the leg are divided into four rather rigid sheaths containing the muscles groups (Figure 7-2). During running, increased blood flow to muscles causes them to swell. Occasionally, the degree of swelling compresses the muscles in the tight deep posterior compartment, causing restriction of blood supply to individual muscle cells and resulting in pain. Many authorities think that this deep posterior compartment syndrome is a major cause of shin splints.

Symptoms and Diagnosis: Pain due to vascular compression develops at the end of a run. It is described as dull, cramping and occasionally associated with numbness or tingling. The toe-off movement of running accentuates this type of shin splint pain.

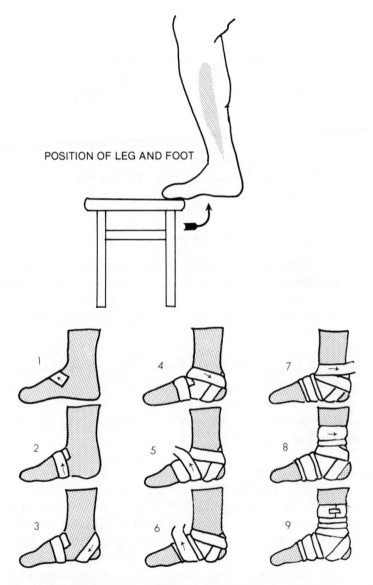

POSITION OF LEG AND FOOT

Use 2½-inch wide x 96-inch long cloth ankle wrap. 1-2. Start on outer side of foot, pull wrap inward under arch. 3. Cross top of foot to outside of ankle and around heel. 4-5. Encircle ankle and pull under inner side of heel. This completes heel lock. 6-9. Complete wrap by applying pressure to lower leg. Secure with clip or tape.

Figure 7-6.   SHIN SPLINT WRAP (REVERSE ANKLE WRAP)

These symptoms usually continue after a runner stops his work-out, persisting for several hours thereafter. Deep posterior compartment shin splints must be distinguished from other types of shin splints (Table 7-1). They will not show up on X ray and bone scans. Local swelling is not usually present.

Comments and Treatment: Some authorities treat this type of shin splint by surgical release of fascia surrounding the posterior compartment. A runner should certainly exclude other possible causes of shin splints before he agrees to this operation. In these instances, a second medical opinion might be helpful.

ANTERIOR COMPARTMENT SYNDROME

Cause: Compartment syndrome may develop in the anterior, lateral, or superficial muscle compartments. These injuries cause acute leg pain rather than chronic shin splints. Compartment syndrome of this type usually develops in untrained runners who cover longer distances than they can handle safely. Inflammation and swelling of muscles develop, resulting in restriction of blood vessels within the tight compartments. Mild cases cause local pain, while more severe swelling may cause extensive muscle damage. The anterior and lateral muscle compartments are the most frequently involved, while the superificial posterior compartment is rarely affected.

Symptoms and Diagnosis: Pain in the involved muscle groups develops during a long distance run. If a runner does not stop early enough, these symptoms can become severe. Pain persists after running is discontinued. Motion of the ankles and toes may cause severe pain. Numbness and tingling of the foot indicates the blood supply to this area is also being restricted.

Note that this injury is an acute problem which occurs in untrained runners engaging in long distance runs.

Comments and Treatments: Be alert to signs of injury when you engage in long distance events, particularly at distances which you have not previously covered. When mild symptoms develop, it is important to stop running. Compartment injury usually disappears rapidly if running is stopped soon enough. If pain continues or increases, seek medical attention immediately. Severe cases require surgical release of the surrounding muscle fascia to relieve the pressure and to allow adequate blood flow to muscle tissue. This must be done within a few hours in order to prevent irreversible muscle destruction.

STRESS FRACTURE OF THE FIBULA

Cause: In the same way that a stress fracture may develop in the tibia, a similar injury can occur in the fibula, the small non-weight-bearing bone that runs along the outer side of the leg.

Symptoms and Diagnosis: The symptoms are similar to those described for stress fracture of the tibia, except that the local pain is felt over the outer side of the lower part of the leg. Stress fractures of the fibula must be differentiated from strains or ligamentous injuries in this area. This diagnosis may be difficult because X rays are usually negative during the first few weeks.

Comments and Treatments: Since the fibula bone is not an important weight-bearing structure, a stress fracture should be treated according to the severity of the symptoms. When the pain is mild, any activity that does not cause undue discomfort is allowed. When pain is severe, however, casting is helpful to allow continued walking with comfort. Running on soft surfaces and adequate cushioning in running shoes also apply here.

8

The Knee

Knee problems are the most common of all running injuries. This joint is vulnerable to injury because of its basic structure. The opposing surfaces within the knee are relatively flat, so the knee is therefore dependent on surrounding ligaments and tendons for support and stability. The knee is designed for to-and-fro motion with only a slight margin for rotation and no allowance for sideway movement.

Basic Structure

The knee is a complex hinged joint joining the femur bone of the thigh and the tibial bone of the leg (Figure 8-1). In front of the knee is the kneecap or patella which slides back and forth in a groove in the femur when the knee is extended and flexed. The kneecap is an important structure used to transfer forces from the powerful quadriceps muscles of the thigh to the leg in order to allow straightening of the knee. It also helps protect the knee joint.

Many of the large thigh muscles pass around the knee, supporting and controlling its motion (Figure 8-2).

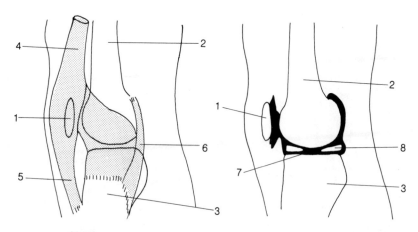

Knee

1 PATELLA

2 FEMUR

3 TIBIA

4 QUADRICEPS TENDON

5 PATELLA TENDON

6 COLLATERAL LIGAMENT

7 JOINT SPACE

8 MENISCUS

9 CARTILAGE

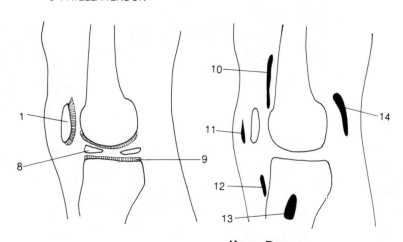

Knee Bursa

10 SUPRAPATELLA

11 PREPATELLA

12 INFRAPATELLA

13 PES

14 POPLITEAL

Figure 8-1. KNEE JOINT

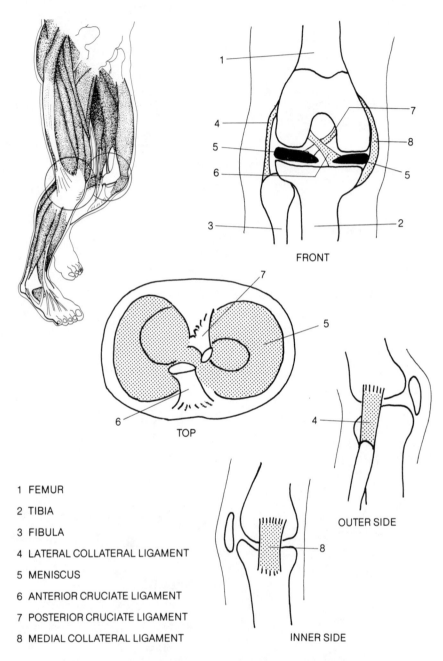

1 FEMUR

2 TIBIA

3 FIBULA

4 LATERAL COLLATERAL LIGAMENT

5 MENISCUS

6 ANTERIOR CRUCIATE LIGAMENT

7 POSTERIOR CRUCIATE LIGAMENT

8 MEDIAL COLLATERAL LIGAMENT

Figure 8-2. LIGAMENTS SURROUNDING KNEE JOINT

Overuse Syndrome

The knee joint is composed of many intricate parts that must function smoothly to produce the fluid motion of running. If any one of these interacting structures becomes inflamed, the delicate balance of the knee is disrupted, and a runner can no longer function without discomfort. This problem very often progresses until he is totally unable to run.

Many runners develop inflammation of one of the structures of the knee, causing a bursitis, tendinitis, synovitis or another type of overuse injury. This can occur when a runner switches to new running terrain such as steep hills or hard pavement, or when he rapidly increases his weekly mileage without allowing the body time to adjust. A runner's knee is usually the weak link that suffers when he overextends himself. It is not uncommon, therefore, for a runner to lament that his training schedule was proceeding according to plan until his knees gave out. Likewise, during the days following extreme stress, such as a marathon race, many runners will suddenly develop a knee injury.

The basic overuse injuries of the knee are tendinitis, bursitis, fasciitis and synovitis.

TENDINITIS

Cause: Any of the tendons that surround the knee can become inflamed from stress (Figure 8-3). Most often, the large quadriceps tendon attaching the quadriceps to the patella, and the patella tendon attaching the patella to the tibia bone are involved. Other common sites include the attachments of the two heads of the calf muscle (gastrocnemius) to the inner and outer sides of the back of the knee; the hamstring tendons where they attach to the back of the fibula; and the pes anserinus tendons at their insertion along the inner front of the tibia.

Symptoms and Diagnosis: Pain and swelling of the tendons over the area of inflammation are usual. Moving the knee causes a grating or sandy feeling over the tendon, indicating inflammation of the tendon as it moves through its sheath. The pain fre-

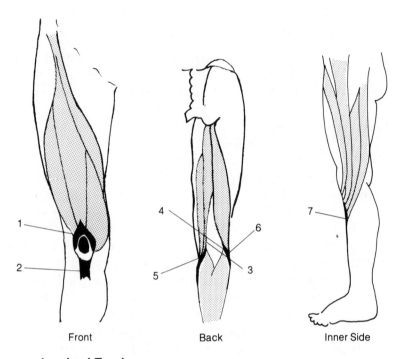

Front	Back

Inner Side

Involved Tendon

1 QUADRICEPS	5 MEDIAL HAMSTRINGS
2 PATELLA	6 LATERAL HAMSTRINGS
3 MEDIAL GASTROCNEMIUS	7 PES ANSERINUS
4 LATERAL GASTROCNEMIUS	

Figure 8-3.   COMMON SITES OF TENDINITIS AROUND KNEE JOINT

quently radiates along a tendon into the body of the muscle. Tendinitis is aggravated by running and improves during rest.

Tendinitis can usually be differentiated from more serious knee injuries by the fact that aside from pain, there is no dysfunction of the knee. In addition, the pain of tendinitis slowly subsides as you warm up, after 15–20 minutes of running.

Comments and Treatment: Treat this injury as you would any tendinitis. Apply heat before and ice after running; take aspirin to help relieve inflammation; and decrease running mileage or allow a few days of complete rest.

BURSITIS

Cause: The knee is surrounded by several bursa that act as lubricating spaces between moving structures (Figure 8-1). When the knee is subject to unaccustomed activity, these bursa can become irritated and inflamed.

Symptoms and Diagnosis: The pain of bursitis may be isolated at the local site of the bursa, or it may produce diffuse knee pain aggravated by the motion of running. Occasionally there is local grating or a scratchy sensation around the bursa. Chronic bursitis may produce marked swelling and fluid collection within the bursa. The most dramatic example of this is "housemaid's knee," a large fluid accumulation in the prepatella bursa in front of the knee.

Bursitis can result in severe dysfuntion of the knee. It may be difficult to localize the cause of pain, and this injury can be confused with other problems within the knee joint. A physician might have to pinpoint the problem.

Comments and Treatment: Mild bursitis usually responds quickly to rest, local ice packs and aspirin therapy. If bursitis becomes chronic, a physician may elect to inject cortisone into the bursa to reduce inflammation. Large fluid accumulations in the prepatella bursa are best treated by removing the fluid with a needle, injecting cortisone into the space and applying a compression wrap.

SYNOVITIS (WATER ON THE KNEE)

Cause: The synovium that lines the knee joint space (see Chapter 4) secretes lubricating synovial fluid. This structure occasionally becomes inflamed and produces large quantities of fluid. Inflammation may result from overuse or from other more serious injuries that irritate the internal structures of the knee.

Symptoms and Diagnosis: The symptoms of synovitis vary from mild diffuse discomfort to severe pain that completely prevents weight bearing. With increased fluid production by the synovium, there is significant diffuse swelling of the knee. It is important to establish the cause of this inflammation. If the synovitis is secondary to an overuse syndrome, it should disappear when running is decreased. When it does not improve with rest, seek medical help to exclude more serious problems.

Comments and Treatment: If the synovitis is associated with overuse, control the inflammation with rest, local ice packs, aspirin and a knee compression wrap (Figure 8-4). Alter your training schedule to allow the knee joint to adapt gradually to increased stress. Sometimes the problem results from relative weakness of the quadriceps muscle. In this case, use quadriceps-strengthening exercises (Chapter 3).

FASCIITIS

The tissue surrounding muscles and loose connective tissue between structures such as ligaments and tendons is called fascia. This tissue can also become inflamed when subject to high levels of stress. Fasciitis usually accompanies tendinitis or bursitis, but it can also be associated with more serious knee problems. Pain may be localized or diffuse in nature. When symptoms do not respond to the usual anti-inflammatory measures, seek medical attention for further evaluation of the knee.

Patella Problems

CHONDROMALACIA

Cause: The term chondromalacia means disintegration of the patella and femoral cartilage surfaces, resulting in uneven rough gliding motion between these structures. Since the kneecap functions under extreme stress from the force generated by the quadriceps muscles, any disruption of the normal smooth gliding motion of this structure will result in cartilage damage. Most commonly, duck-foot walking or abnormal running style causes

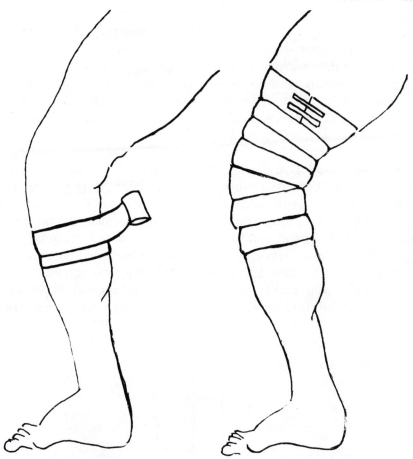

Apply with knee bent approximately 15 degrees. Use 3-inch elastic bandage.
Start below knee and wrap in overlapping pattern ending on lower thigh. Wrap
should be snug, but not too tight.

Figure 8-4.   KNEE COMPRESSION WRAP

chondromalacia. In addition, direct injury or imbalance of thigh
muscle strength can disrupt the usual movement of the kneecap.
Once the patella is damaged, the cartilage surface rapidly becomes rough and irregular. This may lead to pain, discomfort
and swelling within the knee.

Symptoms and Diagnosis: Symptoms associated with chondromalacia usually start as vague deep knee pains with a grating or
crunching sensation felt over the kneecap when it is bent. Dis-

comfort usually increases during activities that stress the pa-
tella-femoral articulation, such as kneeling, walking down stairs
or running down hills. Squatting commonly causes pain. Pressing the kneecap when a runner is lying on a flat surface also
produces pain. Pain is frequently felt along the margin of the
kneecap. With more chronic disease, swelling and tenderness of
the knee can occur (Figure 8-5).

Comments and Treatment: Chondromalacia is a difficult problem to treat; there is no satisfactory cure for it. Therefore, pay
particular attention to early signs of chondromalacia in order to
prevent progression of the symptoms into a more chronic disease. Strengthen the quadriceps muscles with an exercise program (Chapter 3). Have another runner carefully observe your
running style for any idiosyncracy that may be causing chondromalacia, and make every attempt to correct these stylistic
problems. Use only shoes with adequate sole padding to mini-

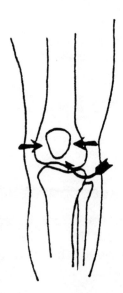

Symptoms include pain and tenderness of the patella and surrounding structures
associated with a grating sensation when you bend your knee.

Figure 8-5. CHONDROMALACIA

mize the shock transmitted to the knees during running. Orthotics, arch supports and wedges often improve this condition.

In addition to weight training, 8–10 aspirin taken daily for a period of up to 2 months sometimes helps in cases of chronic mild chondromalacia. However, be aware of the potential problems associated with aspirin (Chapter 3).

In rare cases of chondromalacia, surgery is indicated. But no operative or medical treatment has proved to be universally successful, and some individuals with this disease may be unable to run.

KNEECAP DISLOCATION

Cause: Occasionally the kneecap is unstable with a tendency to slip out of the normal femoral groove to the side of the knee, causing severe pain, instability and sudden giving way of the knee. Often this problem is associated with weakness of the quadriceps muscle. It may also be due to improper alignment of the kneecap and its tendons with the rest of the muscles of the thigh. Women are much more susceptible to dislocated kneecaps than men (Figure 8-6).

Symptoms and Diagnosis: Runners with this problem are actually able to push the kneecap out of joint with their hands and usually have a history of kneecap popping or slipping to the side. Pain, swelling and spasm of the quadriceps muscles usually follow. Since this problem is frequently inherited, other family members may have similar problems.

Comments and Treatment: A mild condition may respond to quadriceps-strengthening exercises (Chapter 3). If not, or if it is a more chronic condition, it will require surgical treatment to realign the patella and its tendons.

Kneecap dislocation must be adequately treated since chondromalacia frequently develops from damage to the cartilage as it slides in and out of the knee joint during dislocation. Once the kneecap has been stabilized, running can safely be resumed without discomfort.

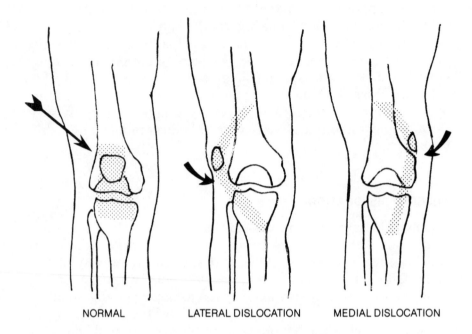

NORMAL   LATERAL DISLOCATION   MEDIAL DISLOCATION

Figure 8-6.   DISLOCATION OF THE PATELLA

Ligament and Cartilage Injuries

ACUTE LIGAMENT INJURIES

Cause: The ligaments that surround the knee joint and provide stability can be acutely injured. Most commonly, runners develop these injuries from falling while they run over irregular terrain or by catching a foot in a hole. Severe stress is placed on the knee, causing injury to the supporting ligaments.

Symptoms and Diagnosis: Following initial injury, the knee may be relatively painfree for several hours. Don't be fooled, however. Curtail further running until the degree of damage can be adequately assessed. In addition to pain, there may be a feeling of instability in the knee following the injury.

Since this injury can be serious, it must be treated by a doctor.

Carefully reconstruct the circumstances of the injury so that a doctor can accurately determine which ligaments have been damaged. For example, if the outside of the knee is struck while falling, the medial collateral ligaments on the inside of the leg will be stretched and injured. With more severe injuries, several ligaments of the knee will be involved. During the first half hour after an injury, the instability of the knee, rather than the pain, will usually be more disabling. A physician will carefully examine the joint to test the integrity of the various ligaments and capsules. X rays may be necessary to see if a bone has been fractured within the knee joint. Other diagnostic studies that may be needed include an arthrogram—an injection of dye into the knee to outline the various structures not usually seen on routine X ray—and arthroscopy—a direct examination of the inside of the knee through a small instrument inserted into the joint.

Comments and Treatment: The treatment of acute ligament injury depends upon the degree of damage. If only a collateral ligament has sustained a sprain, an immobilization splint or cast may be used for 3–6 weeks. More severe injuries that interfere with normal knee functioning usually require surgery and ligament repair. Remember that prolonged immobilization associated with these injuries will cause considerable muscle weakness and atrophy. Once the injury has healed, a muscle-strengthening program will be necessary. We recommend that runners recovering from knee injuries participate in an active swimming program. This allows maintenance of cardiovascular fitness without placing excessive stress on the injured leg.

CHRONIC LIGAMENT INJURY

Cause: Runners frequently suffer from chronic ligament injuries, sometimes referred to as "loose knees." This problem usually arises from an old injury that occurred during a contact sport such as football or wrestling. In these instances, an athlete's knee may remain unstable, either because the injury was not adequately treated at the time, or because the athlete did not engage in a properly supervised muscle-strengthening rehabilitation program. These individuals are often unaware that they have an unstable knee until they begin an active running program.

Symptoms and Diagnosis: Usually there is a feeling of instability in the knee. Moreover, examination of the knee reveals looseness of the ligaments, demonstrated by abnormal side-to-side motion of the knee joint. Runners with this problem often develop swollen sore knees during high mileage training. Synovitis and diffuse tenderness of the knee joint commonly occur at this time.

A runner may be aware that his knee does not function properly and may be able to attribute his disability to an old football injury. Occasionally the knee gives out while a runner participates in special activities such as sprinting or cutting and turning on one leg. Often there is a marked difference in the size of the thigh muscles, the injured leg being smaller than the normal one. Since the injured knee is unable to carry its fair share of the load while running, the normal knee must absorb extra stress. Therefore, a runner will frequently note pain in both knees.

Comments and Treatment: A runner who has chronic instability of the knee should be carefully examined by a physician to assess his ability to withstand the stresses of his running program. Often muscle-strengthening exercises and a program of gradual endurance training cures the problem.

Many ligament injuries can be effectively treated with lightweight metal braces that are specially designed to allow continued running and training while providing adequate support. These braces must be prescribed by a physician and custom fitted and constructed by an orthotist. Over-the-counter elastic knee supports are almost universally ineffective in treating these injuries.

Occasionally, surgery is necessary to reconstruct damaged ligaments. Runners with reconstructed knees, however, are usually unable to compete in long mileage events such as marathons and ultramarathons. Therefore, to avoid misunderstanding and disappointment, you and your surgeon should frankly discuss the reasonable expectations of a surgical procedure.

Many mild cases of instability are aggravated by poor running style and improper foot placement. You can obtain marked improvement of knee symptoms by being fitted with appropriate orthotics and shoe inserts to decrease the abnormal stresses placed on the knee. Your running style should be carefully observed so that the proper shoe insert can be prescribed.

TORN KNEE AND CARTILAGE (MENISCAL TEAR)

Cause: The two knee cartilages or menisci act as shock absorbers in the knee (Figure 8-2). These soft cartilaginous pads can be injured during rotary stress or injuries of the knee which usually occur when you trip or catch the foot on irregular terrain.

Some cases of torn knee cartilage develop without a specific history of injury. These probably result from wear-and-tear degeneration, leading finally to injury of the meniscus.

Symptoms and Diagnosis: Torn knee cartilage can cause a variety of symptoms. Often vague pain is present along either the inside or outside margins of the knee. Sometimes a torn cartilage will slide in and out of the knee joint during bending and stretching, interfering with the normal gliding motion of the opposing surfaces of the femur and tibia. When this occurs, a runner will notice a popping or snapping in the knee, and the knee may temporarily lock until the torn cartilage snaps back into position. Occasionally a torn cartilage will wedge itself permanently in the joint, locking the knee in position. Pain, instability of the knee and swelling are frequently associated with torn cartilage.

When meniscal tears develop gradually, the knee pain progresses slowly as the tear increases in size during repeated stresses of running.

This is another knee problem that requires professional evaluation. In addition to routine examination, the physician will probably take X rays and will perform arthogram and arthoscope evaluation of the knee joint.

Comments and Treatment: When a torn cartilage causes pain, swelling, and clicking or interferes with normal knee motion, it usually must be removed. Often only the torn portion of the cartilage can be excised, leaving the remainder inside the knee to continue its normal functions. Of course, this type of surgery will interfere with the running program for several months.

Some mild cases of torn cartilage can be treated by knee-strengthening exercises (Chapter 3). However, do not embark on this approach until you have been completely evaluated by a physician.

Miscellaneous Knee Problems

JOINT MOUSE (LOOSE CARTILAGE FRAGMENTS WITHIN KNEE JOINT)

Cause: Trauma to the knee joint can chip a small piece of cartilage loose into the joint cavity. Initially this loose body, which is called a joint mouse, causes minimal symptoms. As it floats freely in the knee joint, however, it is nourished by synovial fluid and it grows, eventually becoming so large that it causes significant symptoms and discomfort.

Symptoms and Diagnosis: Symptoms are very similar to those described for torn knee cartilage, including clicking, snapping, swelling, giving way and pain in the knee during running and walking. A runner with a joint mouse may note a round mass in his knee that appears and disappears at various times. Usually, however, the best way to differentiate a joint mouse from a torn cartilage is X-ray evaluation of the knee. The joint mouse will appear as a loose round body within the knee joint.

Comments and Treatment: This loose body can become caught between various surfaces causing damage. It should be removed.

FOREIGN BODY IN THE KNEE

Sometimes a runner will fall and a sharp object such as a splinter or needle will lodge in the knee joint. If this foreign body is not removed, pain, swelling and chronic inflammation of the knee can develop. These symptoms may persist long after the local abrasion from the injury heals. If the runner is not aware that a foreign body has penetrated the knee at the time of an injury, the source of discomfort may be a total mystery. For this reason, X rays are always helpful to exclude unsuspected causes of knee problems.

ARTHRITIS OF THE KNEE

Degenerative or osteoarthritis frequently develops in the knee joint. This may be secondary to an injury; it may reflect improper running form; or it may be an inherited problem. Runners with arthritis of the knees experience symptoms during changes in weather conditions, particularly during cold weather, and during high mileage running. Generalized pain and a grating sensation in the knee are usual. Mild swelling may also be present. Most runners with mild osteoarthritis improve with muscle-strengthening exercises and well-cushioned running shoes. However, some individuals with advanced osteoarthritis are unable to tolerate running and must turn to other activities, such as swimming, to maintain aeorbic fitness.

KNEE INFECTIONS

Infections within the knee joint can occur when a runner falls, cutting the skin or getting a foreign body in the skin or deeper tissues. Most often this infection occurs in the prepatella bursa in front of the kneecap. Swelling, tenderness, redness, local heat in the skin and occasionally fever occur. Chills and fever indicate severe infection. Infection of the knee requires immediate medical attention, for a long-lasting infection will result in irreversible destruction of that joint. A physician will usually drain the pus from the infected area and prescribe antibiotics.

OSGOOD-SCHLATTER'S DISEASE

Fragmentation of the tip of the tibial bone sometimes occurs in children, usually boys, between the ages of ten to fourteen years. It produces pain in front of and immediately below the knee, which is aggravated by running and other strenuous activities. X rays show some enlargement and occasional degeneration of the end of the tibia. This condition does not cause permanent damage, and normal function always returns. Young runners who develop this condition should discuss with their physician the advisability of continuing their running.

BAKER'S CYST

Painless swelling behind the knee joint indicates a local fluid accumulation called a "Baker's cyst." Children most often develop this problem from a congenital weakness of the knee bursa. Baker's cysts of adults are usually associated with diseases of the knee such as arthritis, synovitis, and torn cartilage. A runner with this problem should be examined for underlying diseases of the knee, and X rays of the joint should be taken.

9

The Thigh

Much of a runner's true capacity resides in his thigh. A sprinter gets power from the quadriceps in front of his thigh, while a long distance runner derives most of his strength from the hamstrings in the back of his thigh.

Basic Structure

The thigh (femur) bone connects the hip to the knee (Figure 9-1). Many of the thigh muscles start above the hip and end below the knee joint, so that they move both of these joints. For instance, the rectus femoris—one of the quadriceps muscles—starts in front of the hip and inserts below the knee joint; it flexes the hip forward and straightens the knee joint. These so-called "two-joint muscles" are important for the motion of running. This anatomic arrangement, however, can occasionally complicate a runner's injury. When one joint, such as the knee, is injured, the muscles around that joint become weak. If the same muscle also moves the hip, problems in that joint can occur as a result of the loss of strength of the supporting muscle group.

The muscles of the thigh are divided into three main groups: the anterior muscles, including the quadriceps and sartorious,

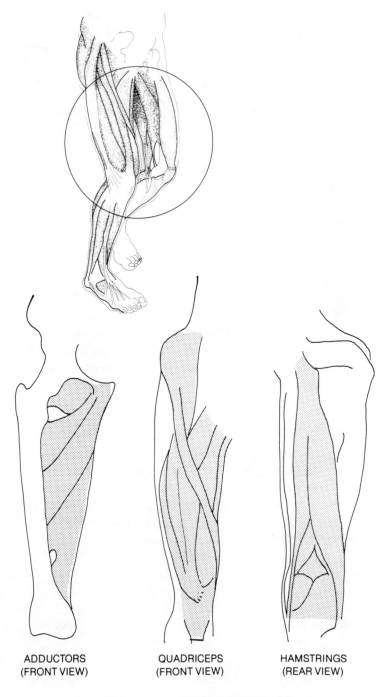

ADDUCTORS
(FRONT VIEW)

QUADRICEPS
(FRONT VIEW)

HAMSTRINGS
(REAR VIEW)

Figure 9-1.   THIGH MUSCLES

which bend the hip forward and straighten the knee; the medial or inner group which bend the knee and bring the hip joint inward; and the posterior group, called the hamstrings, which flex the knee and extend the hip joint backward (Figure 9-1). These muscles attach to various bones of the leg by means of long thick tendons. The quadriceps muscle forms the patella tendon discussed in the chapter on the knee. The medial or adductor muscles attach along the inside shaft of the femur by a broad tendon. The hamstring muscles form tendons that insert on both the inside and outside of the leg; the lateral hamstring attaches along the outside of the knee and on the area of the fibula bone immediately below and to the side of the knee, while the medial hamstrings form a group of tendons that attach along the tibia bone immediately below the inside of the knee.

Thigh Problems

LEG LENGTH DISCREPANCY

Cause: Most individuals are not exactly symmetrical, one foot or hand being slightly larger than the other. In a similar manner, most pairs of femurs are not quite the same length, the normal range being from ¼ to ½ inch difference. Greater differences, however, can result from disturbances in bone growth, congenital problems of the hip and from other less well-recognized causes. This condition is generally called leg length discrepancy, even though it can involve either the leg or the thigh bones. As little a difference as ½ inch will cause uneven stresses on a runner's legs. Most frequently, the knee and hip of the longer leg are subjected to greater forces while running and are injured. Moreover, a runner's pelvis must tilt to compensate for the difference in leg length. This posture produces abnormal stresses on the spine, often resulting in back problems.

Symptoms and Diagnosis: Runners with vague persistent injuries or pain in the knee, hip or back may be suffering from differences in leg length. A diagnosis can be made in several ways. The simplest method for a physician is evaluation of the tip of the pelvic bone when a runner stands barefooted with his feet together. When there is significant leg length discrepancy, one side of the pelvic bone will be higher than the other. You can confirm this observation by standing against a wall and making a mark with a pencil at the top of the pelvic bone on each side. These marks should be the same distance from the floor. More sophisticated measurements can be made with special instruments. Special X rays called orthoroentgenograms measure bone length with an accuracy of a few millimeters.

Comments and Treatment: Runners who have leg length discrepancy of ½ inch or more should place a lift in the sole of the shoe of the shorter leg. Lifts are commercially available, but adequate ones can be made from ¼-inch felt. Sponge rubber does not last as long. Regardless of the difference in leg lengths, the initial lift should be only ¼ inch. If the symptoms improve, add subsequent lifts ¼ inch at a time until the symptoms have disappeared altogether. It is rarely necessary to compensate completely for the discrepancy in leg length, and overcorrection can cause problems. Use the lift in street shoes as well as in running shoes.

SORE MUSCLES (MYOSITIS)

Cause: Runners develop myositis of the thigh muscles following particularly strenuous races or workouts. These aches and pains represent areas of local inflammation and minor injury of the muscle fibers and usually indicate that the runner has pushed himself beyond his limits. For example, soreness of the quadriceps may follow excessive speed or sprint work, while sore hamstrings may develop after an unusually long distance run (see Chapter 4).

Symptoms and Diagnosis: Diffuse aches and pains in the involved muscle groups develop a day after the strenuous activity. Local tenderness is somewhat present. This condition must be distinguished from tendinitis, which is usually much more localized, and from other generalized disease states that can cause muscle soreness.

Comments and Treatment: This overuse syndrome is relatively mild and will clear in a few days. Contrary to most overuse

syndromes, myositis improves more rapidly if running is continued. Therefore, if you awaken with sore muscles on the day
following a particularly hard race, soak in a warm bath or
shower, and then perform stretching exercises followed by easy
walking and jogging. This workout will hasten the disappear-
ance of symptoms. In addition, aspirin taken for 1–2 days will
decrease the inflammation and help alleviate the pain.

PULLED (STRAINED) MUSCLES

Cause: As noted in Chapter 4, a pulled muscle refers to a small
tear or strain injury that results in a muscle cramp. Both the
quadriceps and the hamstring muscles of runners are particularly susceptible to these injuries.

Sprinters can strain either the quadriceps or the hamstring
muscles. Since the quadriceps are essential for generating speed
during sprinting events, these muscles may sometimes be over-
taxed and pulled during the heat of a race. In addition, many
sprinters suffer from muscle imbalance because their quadriceps
are overdeveloped in relationship to their hamstrings. Ideally,
the hamstrings should be 60–70 percent as strong as the quadriceps. Weak hamstring muscles are often overstressed by powerful quadriceps, leading to acute or chronic hamstring injury.

Long distance runners place most training stress on their hamstrings, sometimes overdeveloping this group of muscles. Therefore, fatigue and muscle pull of the weaker quadriceps can occur
during the last miles of a marathon or other long distance race.

Symptoms and Diagnosis: The symptoms of pulled muscles vary
depending upon the severity of the associated injury. A complete muscle tear of the thigh muscles is rare. A pulled hamstring muscle causes pain and inability to bend the knee completely as well as severe pain while trying to straighten that
joint. It is not unusual for a sprinter to pull up lame during a
race as he strains his hamstrings. A pulled quadriceps muscle
causes pain when the knee is flexed. Local spasm and pain over
the involved pulled muscle is common.

Comments and Treatment: Since partial tears can cause insidious symptoms that become progressively more painful, treat

these injuries early with local compression wrap and ice (Figure 9-2). Treat spasm associated with minor muscle pulls by stretching the involved muscle. In the case of the quadriceps bend the knee, while in the event of a hamstring spasm straighten the knee. The pain is often so severe that you will require assistance for this maneuver. Massage of the local muscle spasm helps relieve the pain. If the spasm is relatively mild and disappears with stretching, cautiously resume training. When a spasm recurs, however, a severe muscle pull is possible, and it is best to stop training and treat the local pain with a compression wrap and ice.

Severe muscle pulls should be treated with strict rest for 2 days, combined with local ice therapy to minimize swelling. After this period try light jogging. If pain does not recur, gradually resume workouts. In the case of small partial tears or muscle pulls, complete training activity can usually be resumed in 10—

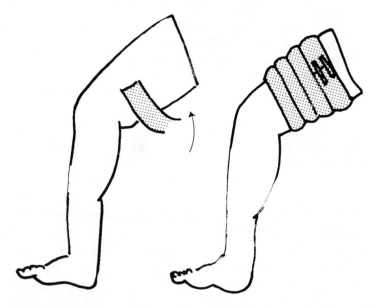

For either quadriceps or hamstring strain. Apply wrap with knee bent approximately 15 degrees. Use 4-inch elastic bandage. Start above knee and wrap in overlapping pattern to end above area of strain. Wrap should be snug, but not too tight.

Figure 9-2.   THIGH COMPRESSION WRAP

14 days. Racing and hard workouts, however, may have to be postponed for 3–4 weeks.

Complete muscle tears must be surgically treated. These types of injuries cause rapid muscle atrophy and weakness and require extensive muscle rehabilitation before resuming normal training activities.

TENDINITIS

Tendinitis of most of the muscles of the thigh occurs where these muscles insert around the knee (see Chapter 8).

10

The Hip

The hip is the strongest and most stable joint of the human body. Therefore, runners injure this structure less frequently than more vulnerable knee, ankle and foot joints. When hip injuries do occur, however, they can totally incapacitate a runner.

Basic Structure

The hip is called a ball-and-socket joint. The head of the femur, or leg bone, is shaped like a ball that fits into the cuplike structure in the pelvic bone, called the acetabulum (Figure 10-1). This arrangement allows the hip to move through an extensive range of motion, including flexion, extension, abduction, adduction and rotation of the leg (Figure 10-2). Large groups of muscles that surround the hip joint allow motion in almost any direction. Surrounding the cup-and-ball arrangement of the head of the femur and the acetabulum is the synovium which secretes lubricating joint fluid. A thick capsule surrounds the joint for protection and stability.

Immediately below the hip joint is a large prominence on the side of the femur bone called the greater trochanter. Thin run-

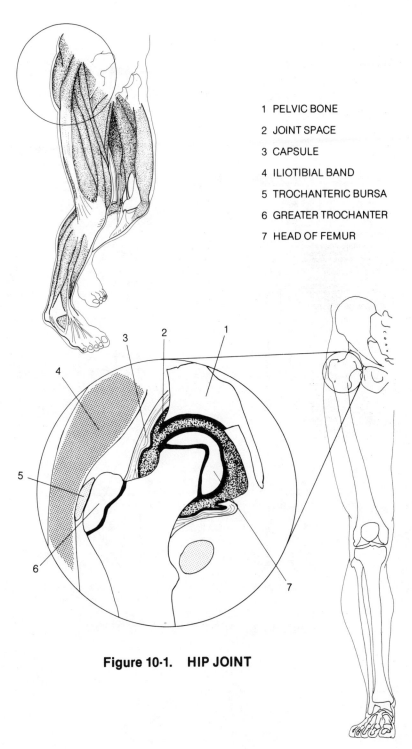

1 PELVIC BONE

2 JOINT SPACE

3 CAPSULE

4 ILIOTIBIAL BAND

5 TROCHANTERIC BURSA

6 GREATER TROCHANTER

7 HEAD OF FEMUR

Figure 10-1.   HIP JOINT

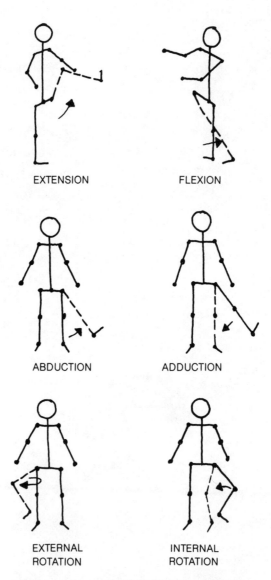

EXTENSION

FLEXION

ABDUCTION

ADDUCTION

EXTERNAL
ROTATION

INTERNAL
ROTATION

Figure 10-2. HIP RANGE OF MOTION

ners can feel this structure on the outer side of their thighs immediately below the hip. The longest ligament in the body, the iliotibial band, runs over the greater trochanter and firmly attaches the pelvis to the tibia. It is one of the principal structures responsible for maintaining the erect posture. A fluid-filled trochanteric bursa lies between the iliotibial band and the greater trochanter, allowing the ligament to glide smoothly over the bone when the hip is flexed and extended.

Injuries

TROCHANTERIC BURSITIS

Cause: This is the most common runners' hip injury. Inflammation of the trochanteric bursa can occur in several ways. Most often, it is an overuse injury, resulting from excessive friction between the iliotibial band and the greater trochanter. Running can cause tightness of the iliotibial band, aggravating trochanteric bursitis. Because the greater trochanter is close to the surface of the skin, this area is susceptible to bruising, another cause of trochanteric bursitis.

Symptoms and Diagnosis: Initially a runner will note pain directly over the greater trochanter. Since running consists of repetitive flexion and extension of the thigh, this activity aggravates trochanteric bursitis as the iliotibial band is repeatedly pulled over the inflamed bursa. Local pressure over the trochanteric bursa may produce pain, and there may be distinct swelling in this area. When the bursitis is the result of an injury or fall, you may note a skin bruise over the greater trochanter.

As trochanteric bursitis becomes more severe, any flexion or extension of the hip becomes extremely painful, and you may be unable to walk. This area may eventually become so sensitive that you cannot lie on your side. Because of its location, trochanteric bursitis can usually be distinguished from synovitis of the hip joint and from capsulitis.

Comments and Treatment: Begin treatment for inflammation—rest, local ice packs and aspirin therapy. In addition, a stretching program to loosen the iliotibial band may help (Figure 10-3). If the bursitis is secondary to an injury, a large amount of local swelling may occur. In this event, accompany ice pack treatment by a local compression wrap to prevent further swelling and accumulation of fluid within the muscle and the bursa. Once the swelling and tenderness begin to subside, resume a schedule of light running.

Cases of chronic bursitis that don't respond to the usual anti-inflammatory measures may require a local injection of cortisone. A runner with persistent pain in this region should consult a physician for further evaluation.

SNAPPING HIP

Cause: Another common problem caused by the iliotibial band is "snapping hip," which is actually a tight snapping over the greater trochanter. Some call this snapping as they flex and extend their hips "dislocating the hip," and it should never be done intentionally because it can irritate the trochanteric bursa, leading to bursitis.

Symptoms and Diagnosis: You may note snapping or popping of the hip while running, especially when the muscles and tendons are stiff. This sensation may or may not be associated with pain, depending upon the degree of associated bursitis.

Comments and Treatment: This condition is usually of no significance unless trochanteric bursitis results. A program of stretching exercises (Figure 10-3) will usually cure it. In rare instances, when snapping hip causes chronic trochanteric bursitis and does not improve from the usual stretching and anti-inflammatory measures, surgical correction to lengthen the band may be necessary.

TRAUMATIC SYNOVITIS

Cause: The synovium lining the inside of the hip joint can react to irritation, injury or infection. Pain, swelling and increased production of fluid in the hip joint are the usual mani-

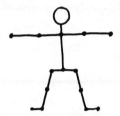

Exercise 1
1. Stand with feet 24 inches apart.
2. Bend to side. Hold 5 seconds.
3. Return to upright.
4. Bend to opposite side.

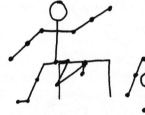
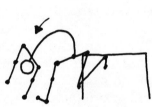

Exercise 2
1. Place leg on table, level with hip.
2. Bend to touch floor. Hold 5 seconds.
3. Alternate sides.

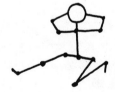
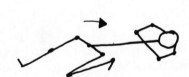

Exercise 3
1. Sit on floor with one leg extended,
   other flexed at side.
2. Lie back on floor. Hold 10 seconds.
3. Return to upright position.
4. Alternate sides.

Figure 10-3.   ILIOTIBIAL LIGAMENT STRETCHING EXERCISES

festations of synovitis. It can be caused by long mileage overuse irritation or can be secondary to a fall that twists or injures the hip. Other cases may occur because of more serious diseases of the hip joint, such as growth abnormalities of young runners and impairment of the hip's normal blood supply.

Symptoms and Diagnosis: Synovitis usually causes the gradual onset of vague hip pain when the hip is rotated inwardly or outwardly. There is some decrease in the normal range of motion of this joint, and you may note inability to run with a full stride because of vague pain and stiffness in the area of the hip. Tenderness deep in the joint is usually felt. These symptoms often progress in severity.

Synovitis of the hip often causes dull aching pain, not severe enough to prevent walking and some degree of running. As a result, runners may delay treating this injury.

Comments and Treatment: Mild overuse synovitis usually disappears after rest and aspirin therapy for a few days. Since more serious conditions can cause hip pain, when symptoms persist they should always be brought to professional medical attention.

CAPSULITIS

The thick fibrous capsule surrounding the hip joint can be injured from overuse, or from overstretching during a fall or slip. This injury causes vague low-grade pain, usually aggravated by running and by rotating the hip inwardly and outwardly. Capsulitis must be differentiated from more serious hip disorders. Treatment consists of anti-inflammatory medications such as aspirin and a limited running schedule. Chronic capsulitis may require deep heat treatment in the form of ultrasound.

GROIN PULL (HIP ADDUCTOR MUSCLE SPRAIN)

Cause: The adductors are a large group of muscles that pull the leg and thigh inward at the hip. These muscles connect the pelvic bone to the inner margin of the femur. Runners most commonly develop groin pulls when these muscles are accidentally overstretched during a sudden fall or slip.

Symptoms and Diagnosis: Following a minor injury, you will note pain in the area of the groin, which is aggravated by outward movement of the thigh. The discomfort is described as a continuous deep ache worsened by walking, running and climbing stairs. These symptoms often improve during rest. Note that the pain often decreases after a warm up and returns following a workout when muscle spasm recurs. The pain may be located only where the muscles attach along the inner margin of the femur, or closer to the pelvic region.

Comments and Treatment: Runners who develop groin strains should begin treatment as soon as injury occurs. Apply ice to help minimize the symptoms, and rest until the initial pain and spasm disappear. After 48 hours, local heat application or soaks in a hot shower or bathtub are recommended (Figure 10-4). Following heat treatment, a thorough range of motion exercises will help decrease spasm. Lying on your back, perform a frog kick motion in three steps:
1. Flex hip by bringing knee upward to the chest.
2. Spread leg to the side.
3. Straighten leg at knee and return to the body.

These exercises should help eliminate the local groin pain. Runners can then resume a slow jogging program, avoiding running tight curves for a few days.

Weakness and atrophy of the muscles involved in this injury occur quite rapidly. Therefore, to prevent recurrent groin strain, include muscle-strengthening exercises as part of the rehabilitation program (see Chapter 3).

ARTHRITIS OF THE HIP

Cause: Degenerative arthritis often involves the hip joint. This wear-and-tear roughening of joint cartilage can be the result of an old injury such as a hip dislocation from an automobile accident. Other causes may include inherited instability of the hip,

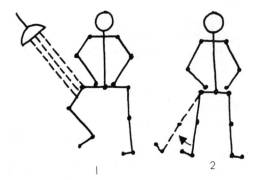

Exercises performed in warm shower 1. Flex knee and rotate hip outward. 2. With knee locked, extend leg to side.

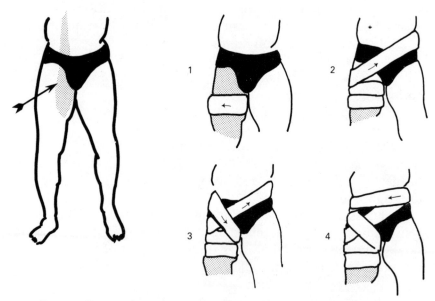

Compression wrap for groin support 1. Using a 6-inch elastic bandage, encircle thigh 8 inches below groin. 2. Encircle waist. 3. Pull wrap down and around groin. 4. Finish wrap with a second loop around the waist. Secure with tape or clips.

Figure 10-4.   GROIN STRAIN

obesity, growth disturbances and leg discrepancy, each of which causes abnormal stresses on the hip joint.

Symptoms and Diagnosis: Irregular cartilage surfaces within a degenerative hip may produce pain and intermittent swelling of that joint. A runner with degenerative arthritis may note gradual onset of vague, constant hip pain not associated with a specific level or intensity of training. He may have a history of one of the problems just described. Arthritis increases during changes in weather, particularly during cold damp seasons.

It usually takes years for degenerative arthritis to produce significant symptoms. You may note decreased range of motion of one hip joint, sometimes associated with a crunching or grinding sensation within the hip. An X ray of the hip is necessary to establish the cause of hip pain and to assess the degree of damage associated with degenerative arthritis.

Comments and Treatment: Many runners with mild degenerative arthritis benefit from a training program. Running helps you lose weight, thus decreasing the stress on hip joints. There is absolutely no truth to the myth that running hastens degenerative changes. In fact, some studies indicate that runners have a lower incidence of degenerative arthritis than do nonrunners. Those runners who do have mild degenerative arthritis can experience mild flare-ups of pain, best treated with aspirin and a few days of rest.

Persons with severe cases of degenerative arthritis may be unable to engage in a running program. The hip simply will not tolerate running. Swimming is an excellent aerobic activity to establish cardiovascular fitness for these would-be athletes.

STRESS FRACTURE OF THE NECK OF THE FEMUR

Cause: A stress fracture of the neck of the femur is a serious overuse injury. Fortunately, it is also relatively uncommon.

Symptoms and Diagnosis: Beginning runners are most prone to this injury, which causes a deep constant ache in the hip joint, aggravated by running and relieved *only* by lying down and taking the weight off the hip. It usually afflicts those who are relatively unfit, slightly obese and have overextended their training programs. A physician may request X rays and bone scans to diagnose this fracture.

Comments and Treatment: This injury represents a potentially serious and incapacitating problem. Stress fractures can progress to complete break of the bone, requiring surgical intervention. Treatment should be supervised by a physician. Crutches are recommended for several weeks to prevent weight bearing on the injured bone. Following X ray evidence of healing, gradually increase activity until complete recovery occurs.

CONGENITAL HIP PROBLEMS

Cause: There are several conditions that occur early in life which may lead to later problems of the hip joint. These include dislocation of the hip at birth, changes in the normal growth of the hip joint (Perthes' disease), slipped femoral growth plate and traumatic dislocation previously described.

Many conditions causing injury to the hip in childhood result in degenerative arthritis of the adult hip. Therefore, when a child develops persistent pain of the hip, consult a physician.

Symptoms and Diagnosis: *Perthes' disease* is due to a temporary disturbance in the blood supply and normal growth area of the head of the femur. This usually occurs in children between the ages of five and ten and affects only one hip. The child will complain of pain in the groin or thigh and will limp. The severity of this problem is quite variable, and parents should seek the advice of a physician in order to minimize permanent damage.

Slipped capital femoral epiphysis usually affects teenage runners between the ages of twelve to seventeen. They may develop pain in the hip and knee, associated with a limp. This can be due to a slippage or upward sliding of the neck and shaft of the femur. Immediate medical attention is indicated to prevent damage. X rays confirm this diagnosis. Since this condition can result in leg length discrepancies, treatment requires surgical correction.

Note that the hip problems just discussed are not *caused* by running, and there is no evidence that strenuous activity such as running is in any way harmful or detrimental to growing children. On the contrary, endurance sports may be quite beneficial to a growing cardiovascular system.

11

Miscellaneous Injuries

In addition to those injuries discussed in the preceding chapters, runners often encounter other problems and several miscellaneous injuries, including lacerations, dog bites and frostbite.

THE BACK AND NECK

The back is a complex structure particularly susceptible to injuries. Since most back problems are aggravated by poor muscle tone and obesity, running often improves symptoms associated with back injuries. Occasionally, however, running itself seems to aggravate the problem. While there is tremendous individual variation in this regard, there does seem to be a distinct "runners' back."

Basic Structure

The bones that form the spine are called vertebrae (Figure 11-1). Between these bones are resilient cushions of connective tissue called discs which act to cushion the spine. Joints between

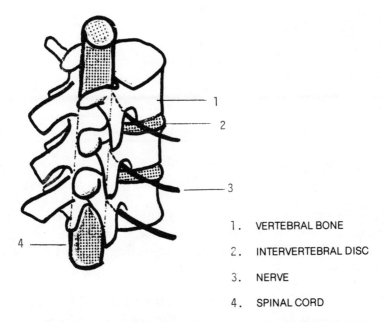

1. VERTEBRAL BONE
2. INTERVERTEBRAL DISC
3. NERVE
4. SPINAL CORD

Figure 11-1. VERTEBRAL BONES AND SPINAL CORD

the vertebrae permit movement and flexibility of the spine. The spinal cord, which carries nerves from the brain to the rest of the body, runs through a protective canal in the vertebrae. Individual nerves from the spinal cord leave the canal through channels between individual vertebra. Along the sides of the vertebrae are strong muscles, called paraspinal muscles, which support the spine and allow appropriate movement. The human spine is usually curved in the low back in a slight swayback, called lordosis.

Injuries to the back can result from damage to the vertebrae or intervertebral discs, abnormal shape of the spine such as exaggerated swayback configuration, poor posture, weakness of the abdominal muscles, excessive strain on the paraspinal muscles and obesity. In many instances, back problems become chronic as degeneration and arthritis of the vertebrae and the joints of the spine develop. These abnormalities often cause irritation or pressure on nerves as they exit from the spinal cord, causing pain and occasional weakness of the muscles supplied by the nerves. In addition, the intervertebral discs lose elasticity with aging, making them particularly prone to injuries.

Back injuries of particular importance to runners usually involve the lower half of the spine in the region called the low back or lumbosacral spine. These injuries include low back sprain, chronic low back sprain, ruptured or slipped discs, scoliosis and spondylosis.

Back and Neck Problems

LOW BACK SPRAIN

Cause: This injury is usually the result of sprain of the paraspinal muscles from unaccustomed stress, such as lifting or twisting. Tendons and ligaments surrounding the vertebrae may also be injured.

Symptoms and Diagnosis: Back sprain usually develops suddenly during unnatural stress on the back, causing a sudden twinge or pulling sensation in the injured area. This injury, however, may develop several hours after unusually heavy exertion as the paraspinal muscles gradually go into spasm. Because the spasm causes considerable pain, this injury is usually quite disabling.

This problem must be distinguished from more serious injury such as a ruptured disc. Symptoms of numbness, tingling or weakness in the back, legs or buttocks suggests more serious injury requiring medical attention.

Comments and Treatment: Treat back sprain with decreased activity or complete bed rest and aspirin therapy until symptoms improve. Pain symptoms often improve dramatically following local moist heat treatment. Massage of the rigid muscle spasm is also soothing. Pain relief and muscle-relaxing drugs are often prescribed by physicians. Most cases of simple back sprain clear up after a few days of rest and local heat, but if the symptoms do not improve after 7–10 days of rest, medical attention should certainly be sought.

CHRONIC LOW BACK SPRAIN

Cause: Some individuals are susceptible to recurrent sprains of the back. In many instances, there is some underlying cause such as an abnormal shape of the spine, a tilting pelvis, or unusual posture or running form. This injury may occur with or without an episode of heavy lifting or undue back stress.

Symptoms and Diagnosis: Recurrent episodes of spasm of the paraspinal muscles, especially when not associated with unusual activity, suggest chronic low back sprain. Be careful to distinguish it from more serious problems. Numbness, tingling or weakness of the back or leg muscles suggests ruptured disc or arthritis.

Comments and Treatment: Chronic low back sprain is a particularly disabling injury that can often be traced to an underlying problem predisposing you to this injury. For this reason, careful medical examination and evaluation including X rays is usually necessary. Runners with chronic low back sprain should seek the advice of a physician.

When complete medical evaluation reveals no detectable abnormalities, there may be subtle muscle imbalances related to posture, running form and what is loosely termed "weak back." These cases often respond to a program of back exercises to strengthen the paraspinal muscles, to correct improper posture of the spine, and to strengthen the abdominal muscles in order to help the paraspinal muscles support the body. These exercises are illustrated in Figure 11-2 and should be performed daily. In addition, swimming is an excellent exercise for individuals who suffer from back problems.

SLIPPED OR RUPTURED DISC

Cause: The intervertebral disc between vertebrae occasionally ruptures out of its normal location to press on the spinal canal, causing damage of the nerves. This condition results from a combination of factors, including degeneration of the disc with age,

back exercises (flexion)

3 sets of 10, with rest in between each 10. Exercises should be performed daily, and should not exceed 3 x 10 at any one session. However, the exercises may be repeated several times per day, staying with the 30 count each time.

1. flat on back, hands over head

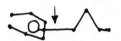

1. Tighten abdomen and buttocks, pushing back on floor.
2. Hold for a count of 3.
3. Relax.
4. Repeat 30 times, resting after each set of 10.

2. flat on back, hands over head again

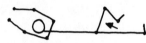

1. Bend knee to chest while stretching opposite leg.
2. Bring knee back down.
3. Alternate.
4. Repeat 30 times, resting after each set of 10.

3. flat on back, hands at side

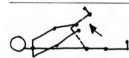

1. Grab knee and pull to chest.
2. Bring knee back down.
3. Alternate.
4. Repeat 30 times, resting after each set of 10.

4. flat on back, hands at side again

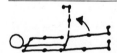

1. Raise leg straight, with knee stiff.
2. Bring leg down slowly.
3. Alternate.
4. Repeat 30 times, resting after each set of 10.

5. flat on back, hands on chest

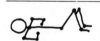

1. Press hands against chest, attempt to sit up.
2. Hold for 5 seconds.
3. Repeat 30 times, resting after each set of 10.

6. flat on back, hands behind neck

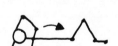

1. Hands in back of neck, pull head to knees.
2. Hold.
3. Return slowly.
4. Repeat 30 times, resting after each set of 10.

note: If difficult, press hands into abdomen and attempt to sit up. Do not jerk!

7. standing up, against a wall

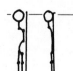

1. Stand erect, back to wall.
2. Tilt pelvis so that back is actually against wall.
3. Hold.

Figure 11-2.

improper posture and direct or recurrent injury to the spine. Because a ruptured disc causes pressure on the nerves of the spinal cord, it is an extremely serious injury that requires expert medical care.

Symptoms and Diagnosis: A ruptured disc usually causes severe pain in the back often associated with numbness and tingling radiating from the back down into the buttocks and legs. The pain may be so dramatic that you are totally unable to stand or move. Occasionally, less severe degrees of ruptured disc cause the same symptoms, though chronic or intermittent and less extreme.

Runners with this condition must seek the care of a physician. In addition to routine X rays of the spine, a procedure called a myelogram may be performed to diagnose slipped disc. This entails injection of dye into the spinal canal to identify the exact location of the disc pressing against the nerve cord.

Comments and Treatment: Mild cases of ruptured disc usually respond to bed rest, local heat, pain relievers and muscle relaxants used for muscle sprains. It may take several weeks for complete recovery to occur. Once the initial pain and discomfort have disappeared, supervised exercise programs are indicated. Those individuals who do not respond to conservative treatment may require surgical removal of the offending disc. Since recovery from this operation requires several months, runners with slipped discs should comply fully with the recommendations for conservative rest therapy. Running with a ruptured disc is an extreme folly that can lead to catastrophic complications.

CURVATURE OF THE SPINE (SCOLIOSIS)

Cause: Many individuals develop a "crooked spine" due to hereditary or growth problems. This deformity is much more common in girls than boys and usually becomes evident during the ages of ten to eighteen.

Symptoms and Diagnosis: Initially, curvature of the spine causes no symptoms. Close examination by parents or doctor will reveal a serpentine or crooked configuration of the spine. With time, other diseases of the spine such as recurrent back sprain and slipped disc may develop.

Comments and Treatment: Careful medical assessment of the degree of deformity will determine the appropriate treatment. Most cases require only observation. Young runners with mild scoliosis can participate in running programs without difficulty. More severe cases, however, and progressive deformity may require braces and back-strengthening exercises to prevent difficulties. Early therapy can prevent deformity and extensive surgery.

SPONDYLOSIS

Cause: Some individuals are born with a defect in the back of the vertebral bone. This condition is called spondylosis.

Symptoms and Diagnosis: While many people with spondylosis have no symptoms, others may develop recurrent back problems. Individuals with chronic low back pain, sprain and slipped discs should be evaluated for this defect which will appear on X rays of the spine.

Comments and Treatment: Treatment of spondylosis depends on the degree of discomfort. Those individuals without any symptoms can participate in all activities including running, while those with symptoms may occasionally not be able to run. Swimming is an alternative exercise. If spondylosis is associated with instability of the spine, it may require surgical treatment.

RUNNER'S BACK

Sometimes beginning runners will note the development of back pain. While some runners may have a previous history of back problems, others will experience this discomfort for the first time. Running causes extra stress on the paraspinal muscles which may unmask a subtle imbalance or deformity of the spine. Other instances are the result of leg length discrepancies or similar problems that cause a pelvic tilt and unusual stress on the paraspinal muscles.

Runners who develop back pain should carefully analyze their symptoms according to the diagnoses outlined above. Those with chronic back sprain or symptoms suggestive of a slipped disc should be completely evaluated by an experienced physician. Once the usual causes of back problems are excluded, particular attention should be given to running form, asymmetry of gait, leg length discrepancies, and running conditions. The sloping asphalt of roads frequently causes road runners to run with one foot higher than the other, resulting in muscular imbalance of the paraspinal muscles as the pelvis tilts. In a similar manner, running on tight turns of a small track will cause abnormal stresses on your back as you constantly lean toward the inside leg. Runners with back problems should try running on soft surfaces and select shoes with particularly well-cushioned soles. Avoid long runs on hard surfaces and over irregular terrain.

Most back problems actually improve following the institution of a running program. Running strengthens the paraspinal muscles and is usually not associated with twisting or other stressful movements of the spine. For this reason, many individuals who develop back problems from sports such as tennis turn to running as an alternative exercise.

STIFF NECK

Runners frequently develop stiff necks. In some instances, this problem is related to degenerative arthritis of the cervical (neck) spine, which causes irritation of local nerves supplying the muscles in the neck. Movement of the neck or exercise such as running occasionally aggravates this nerve root irritation, and the paraspinal muscles in the neck develop spasm which produces pain. Occasionally the reasons for neck pain are not clear. Some authorities theorize that evaporation of sweat chills the exposed neck area, resulting in muscle stiffness.

Treatment of stiff neck consists of medication such as aspirin to relieve pain and immobilization of the neck with a soft cervical collar. In addition, local heat packs and massage help relieve muscle spasm.

Individuals with mild degenerative arthritis of the cervical spine often report recurrent episodes of stiff neck. These flare-ups are best treated with the above measures. Wearing a soft cervical collar throughout the day and at night will speed recovery.

When neck spasm seems to result from evaporation of sweat and exposure to cold drafts, wear a towel muffler wrapped around the neck while running to minimize the problem.

MINOR INJURIES

ABRASIONS AND SUPERFICIAL LACERATIONS

These small injuries to the skin are best treated by cleaning with soap and water. Treat local bleeding with pressure applied with a sterile dressing. Then clean the wound of all foreign matter and treat with 70% alcohol and iodine containing antiseptic solution. A loose sterile dressing should be taped in place and changed daily so that the wound may be carefully inspected. Redness, swelling or pus indicates the development of infection. The inflamed area should be soaked in lukewarm water for 15 minutes every few hours. Apply the soaks with a clean wet washcloth, or submerge the wound in a basin of water. If the infection does not respond in 24 hours, consult a doctor. If all goes well, a wound may be exposed to air within 48 hours when a scab forms. Because scabs that form over joints often break down as the result of motion and pulling of the skin, wear a dressing coated with petroleum jelly over this type of skin injury.

NIPPLE IRRITATION AND ABRASION

Runners sometimes develop irritation or abrasion of their nipples from friction of their skin against their clothes. Nylon and synthetic running shirts are more likely to cause this problem than are cotton T-shirts. Women may prevent nipple injury with a soft bra and liberal application of petroleum jelly or talcum powder. Men should use petroleum jelly or Band-Aids to protect their nipples. Because painful nipples often develop during a long distance race, such as a marathon, it is wise to prevent the problem by covering sensitive nipples before a race begins.

DOG BITES

Unfortunately runners frequently suffer dog bites. These injuries are usually puncture wounds, although they sometimes result in ragged lacerations. Thoroughly wash the wound with soap and water and cover with a sterile dressing. Many animal bites become infected. Deep wounds or wounds that become red, swollen or pussy should be treated by a doctor. Whenever possible, the dog should be caught and observed for rabies which is still a hazard in certain parts of the United States.

CINDER BURNS

When a runner falls on a cinder track, the resulting scratches and abrasions are usually contaminated by cinders. Remove this imbedded debris by washing thoroughly with soap and water. Sometimes a small stiff brush is helpful. The wound will bleed during brushing, but this helps remove cinders and dirt. Once a wound is thoroughly cleaned, apply an antiseptic solution. Dress the wound with antibacterial ointment to help loosen any imbedded cinders.

PUNCTURE WOUNDS

Runners who run barefoot can sustain deep puncture wounds of the feet. Spiked track shoes are another common cause of this type of injury. Punctures can carry dirt and bacteria deep under the skin, resulting in serious infections of soft tissue and bone (osteomylitis). Thoroughly wash these injuries with soap and water and cover with a loose dressing. Continued pain, swelling or redness should be brought to medical attention. A doctor may decide to explore the injured area for any trapped foreign material, and he may recommend antibiotics. Puncture wounds are a common site of tetanus infection (see Chapter 13).

FROSTBITE

Exercising muscles generate considerable heat from body metabolism. For this reason, runners are usually comfortable at low environmental temperatures. However, the nose, chin, ears, fingers and penis (see Chapter 17) are susceptible to frostbite injury. Whenever environmental temperatures are below freezing, frostbite is possible, although it usually does not develop until temperatures are much lower. A combination of wind and cold is particularly dangerous since these two elements combine to produce a wind-chill factor, greatly enhancing the danger of cold-induced injury.

Initial symptoms of frostbite include numbness and a tingling sensation. The involved skin appears white.

Emergency treatment consists of warming the involved skin. Runners should cover the injured site immediately and seek a warm shelter. Simply covering the involved nose or ear with a scarf or gloved hand will often provide adequate warmth to relieve frostbite symptoms. Avoid rubbing the skin since this will cause damage. If possible, rapidly warm the involved area with lukewarm water. Severe frostbite should be treated by a physician.

It's far better to take a few preventive steps, and, in fact, prevention of frostbite is a necessity among those runners who live in cold climates. Ears should be covered with a wool cap. A ski mask is sometimes necessary to protect sensitive facial areas. Gloves and socks are recommended to prevent frostbite of the digits. Although toes are normally the most susceptible area to frostbite, runners seem to develop cold injury of these digits less frequently than the general population. The motion of running and the friction between running shoes and feet appear to offer some protective value. Nylon running gear is a better barrier to wind than is cotton and helps eliminate the wind-chill factor.

12

The Skin

A runner's skin is his most vulnerable body organ. Sun, wind, heat, cold, air pollution, infections and allergies all take their toll. Preventive skin care, probably the most neglected of a runner's medical needs, will help avoid "runners' skin" and the stereotype of a wrinkled old man in a young healthy body.

Basic Structure and Function

The skin is the largest and one of the most important of the body's organs. It is composed of two layers: the outer, called the epidermis; and the inner, the dermis (Figure 12-1). The outermost layer of the epidermis is continually sloughed off as new skin is formed in the inner epidermal layers. The epidermis contains the pigment cells responsible for the color of the skin. The dermis contains hair follicles, sweat glands, nerve endings and a rich network of small blood vessels. The skin is thicker on those parts of the body exposed to pressure such as the palms and soles.

The skin is a barrier to protect the body from bacteria, viruses and harmful chemicals in the atmosphere. It conserves vital

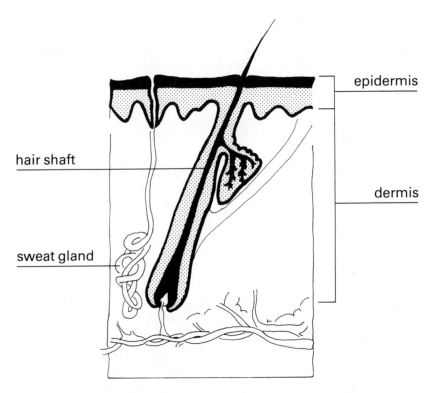

The outer layer, the epidermis, regenerates new cells and thickens at sites of chronic friction. The dermis contains sweat glands and blood vessels important for body temperature regulation.

Figure 12-1.   SKIN

fluids, preventing the body from becoming dehydrated. One of the most important functions of the skin is temperature regulation. During hot weather, blood is shunted to the skin where heat is lost by radiation. In addition, sweat glands produce perspiration which cools the body as it evaporates. In cold weather, blood is directed away from the skin to conserve body heat. This insulating factor allows the skin temperature to drop several degrees while the inner body temperature remains normal.

Alterations During Running

The most important function of the skin during exercise is to dissipate body heat produced by the muscles' metabolic processes. This is extremely important in preventing the body from overheating during long runs, particularly in hot humid weather. This function is discussed in Chapter 18.

During training, adaptation occurs which increases the amount of sweat produced as well as the amount of salt in the sweat. These changes allow more efficient cooling of the body during exercise and are discussed more fully in Chapter 18.

Skin Problems

Of all the body's organs, a runner's skin probably takes the most abuse. Year-round exposure to the elements—sun, wind, heat and cold—causes premature aging, freckles, dryness and even skin cancer. Skin on runners' feet is frequently afflicted with a variety of infections and allergic reactions. Fortunately most of these problems are avoidable, and recognition of potential dangers coupled with preventive measures will avoid serious discomfort and disabling disease.

SUNLIGHT—A DANGEROUS FRIEND

Ultraviolet rays in natural sunlight cause sunburn, as well as tanning of the skin. While the sun is one of the great pleasures of outdoor running, the danger of ultraviolet rays is considerable. Some of the problems it causes are:

1. *Sunburn.* Most runners have tanned skin from daily exposure to sunlight. They are, therefore, not likely to be sunburned unless there is a drastic change in the amount of sun exposure.

2. *Aging of the skin.* Wrinkles are the skin's way of growing old. The same ultraviolet light that tans skin also wrinkles it, and because runners spend more time in the sun, their skin is more wrinkled than people of the same age. Fair-skinned people are most susceptible to this problem, but no one is completely immune. An honest look in the mirror will reveal excessive dry-

· ness and wrinkles. Weather-beaten, freckled, tanned, dry, wrinkled skin is a trademark of veteran runners and could properly be termed "runners' skin." Premature aging of the skin can be greatly minimized by blocking out dangerous ultraviolet rays with lotions called sunscreens, available in drugstores. Look for ingredients such as para-aminobenzoic acid (PABA), benzophenone and cinnamate. They all work effectively. Regular suntan lotion does not screen out dangerous ultraviolet rays. In addition, replacement of skin's natural oils with moisturizing cream or baby oil will help fight wrinkles.

3. *Freckles and sun spots.* Freckles are areas of dense pigmentation in the skin. They increase with exposure to sunlight. In addition, rough reddish-brown or gray growths frequently develop on sun-exposed areas. They are called solar or actinic keratosis. Most usually grow slowly, but some develop into skin cancer. Any abnormal growth on the skin should be brought to the attention of a dermatologist (skin specialist). Solar keratosis can develop into cancer and should be removed either by surgery or with a cream containing 5-fluorouracil, an anticancer drug.

4. *Skin cancer.* Risk of skin cancer increases with exposure to ultraviolet light of the sun. Once again, this is most common in fair-skinned people. When an ulcer of the skin does not heal, one should suspect skin cancer and consult a dermatologist. Runners over the age of forty should be particularly aware of this danger. Fortunately, skin cancer is almost always curable if treated within a reasonable period of time. Cancers are removed by a simple surgical excision. Larger lesions are treated with radiation therapy.

5. *Photoallergic reactions.* Rays of the sun will sometimes react with substances on the skin such as cosmetics, lipsticks, deodorant soaps, after-shave lotions and ointments, to cause a severe allergic reaction similar to a painful sunburn. This may also occur when you take certain medications such as sulfa, phenothiazide tranquilizers and oral medications for diabetes. The disease is allergic, and therefore not everyone who uses these substances will develop a reaction.

Redness, swelling and even blistering of exposed parts of the body after a relatively small dose of sunlight suggests a photoallergic reaction. Like sunburn, there is usually a clear demarcation line where clothing protects the skin from direct sunlight. An alert runner can diagnose a photoallergic reaction by being aware of the problem.

Photoallergic reactions will clear when the runner stops using the offending medication or cosmetic. Very severe reactions may require temporary treatment with cortisone cream or pills. These must be prescribed by a physician.

Most runners plan to run for the rest of their lives. That means many years of exposure to dangerous ultraviolet light. Be smart about the sun. Enjoy it, but don't punish your skin. Use of sunscreens and moisturizing lotions is medically intelligent and certainly not sissy stuff.

SKIN INFECTIONS (ATHLETE'S FOOT, JOCK ITCH, BOILS AND OTHER BUGS)

Millions of bacteria and fungi normally live on the skin. When excessive moisture, chafing, scrapes, pressure points from shoes, or blisters weaken the skin, the microorganisms (bugs) frequently take advantage of the situation to cause infection. Other bugs accumulate on locker-room floors, showers, dirty towels, socks and jocks and are picked up by careless runners who do not use proper hygiene. Pus and fever usually mean bacterial infection. A sample of pus or skin can be sent to a laboratory to identify the type of bacteria.

1. *Athlete's foot, jock itch and rashes* in body creases (intertrigo) are usually caused by *fungal infection.* Tinea and candida (monilia) are the two types of fungi responsible for these lesions. Their rashes may be identical, but because tinea and candida fungi are treated differently, sometimes it is necessary for a doctor to distinguish one from the other by examining a scraping of skin under a microscope. Small red patches in body creases spread outward with pinhead blisters or scales at the margins. Athlete's foot develops as small blisters, scaling, redness or degeneration of the skin between the toes, webs or soles of the feet. These infections may be itchy or painful.

Runners can self-treat most cases of suspected athlete's foot and other fungal infections. Ointments or powders such as Tinactin, Halotex and Micatin will cure mild cases of either candida or tinea. Coaches and trainers frequently use Whitfield's ointment (benzoic acid and salicylic acid). Soaking the feet in Castellani's carbol-fuchsin solution (available in drugstores) will bring immediate relief for severe cases. Resistant cases that don't respond to these measures require a doctor. He will treat tinea with griseofulvin pills and candida with nystatin cream. Severe cases in the rectal or vaginal area may require oral nystatin. Almost every runner has experienced fungal infections of the foot. Remember that fungi love damp skin, and the best prevention is careful drying and powdering of the feet.

2. *Toenail infection* with tinea fungus leads to yellow discoloration and heaped-up matter under the nail. The end result is rough, irregular nails that rub against shoes and cause considerable pain and blister formation. It usually takes several weeks of griseofulvin pills to cure toenail fungus.

3. *Impetigo* is an itchy rash caused by streptococcus or staphylococcus bacteria. These infections are very contagious, and runners usually pick them up from contaminated towels, locker-room benches or shower floors. Epidemics of impetigo may infect an entire track team. Small blisters form on the face, arms, body or legs. Pus or honey-colored crust oozes when the blister is opened, and infection spreads to adjacent skin. This infection usually itches.

Impetigo and other bacterial infections often require antibiotics. Impetigo usually responds to washing with soap and water and application of antibiotic ointment. Severe cases require penicillin pills. Epidemics of streptococcal impetigo may lead to glomerulonephritis, a serious kidney disease. When several team members develop impetigo, all locker-room facilities should be meticulously cleaned, as should all shared equipment such as socks, jocks and uniforms.

4. *Pyoderma* is also a bacterial infection due to streptococcus or staphylococcus. These infections frequently develop in areas of skin previously damaged by fungal infection or allergic dermatitis. Treatment is similar to impetigo. Antibiotic pills are frequently required.

5. *Boils* are deep collections of pus usually caused by staphylococcus bacteria. Poor hygiene of the feet, negligent care of

blisters, fungal infections or minor abrasions may lead to a boil. These are dangerous infections because staphylococcus can enter the bloodstream and cause serious "blood poisoning."

Boils begin as tender red spots and gradually develop into large pimples or pus pockets which may open and drain thick white or green pus. Fever indicates serious infection.

Soak boils in warm water. They usually require treatment with antistaphylococcal pills (Dicloxacillin) and may have to be surgically drained. Never squeeze a boil or run with one on the foot. Bacteria may be forced into the bloodstream.

6. *Paronychia* is an infection of the nail cuticle with candida fungus or staphylococcus bacteria. Pressure from running shoes or improper nail clipping may cause this problem. Soak foot in warm tap water for 15 minutes three times a day. Apply nystatin cream for candida or take Dicloxacillin pills for staphylococcal infection.

7. *Cellulitis,* painful red swelling of the skin, is due to streptococcus or staphylococcus bacteria that invade the skin through small cuts or other damaged sites. Infection spreads rapidly up the leg. Chills and fever are common. This is a very dangerous condition, potentially life threatening. In addition, it may lead to permanent damage of the vascular drainage of the leg and chronic swelling. Antibiotics are mandatory and hospitalization is sometimes necessary.

8. *Vincent's disease* is a painful, swollen mouth due to bacterial infections. Runners may develop this problem by sharing contaminated drinking cups or contaminated "sucking towels" frequently present on the track. Candida infections of the mouth can develop in the same way. Sore, red mucous membranes with blisters on the inside of the mouth suggest Vincent's disease, while patches on the tongue or mucous membranes indicate candida.

Vincent's disease is treated with penicillin mouth wash. Nystatin solution is used to treat candida of the mouth.

9. *Herpes infection* (fever sores and other painful blisters). Herpes simplex virus causes painful blisters of the skin. This infection follows two clinical patterns. Some individuals note fever sores or blisters in the area of the lips or nose while suffering from other infections such as the common cold, or after ex-

posure to sunlight. In these cases the herpes virus lives in the skin in a dormant state for the whole life of the individual. For reasons that are not entirely clear, sunlight and infections cause the virus to multiply, resulting in painful fever blisters. These blisters then subside within a week or two, only to recur again at some future time. Fever sores can be particularly troublesome to runners who are exposed to large amounts of sunlight. This type of herpes infection is not contagious.

Pain from herpes infection usually develops before a cold sore is evident. A skin lesion then develops within 24 hours. Over the next few days the blister will mature, then rupture, leaving a scab that slowly disappears. The whole process usually takes a few days to 2 weeks. There is usually no fever or swelling of the lymph glands or other signs of body infection. To minimize the risk of developing this infection, use a sunscreen cream when ultraviolet light-induced herpes is involved, and practice good hygiene. Unfortunately, there is no specific cure for herpes simplex virus infections. Occasional early treatment with a medication called idoxuridine will minimize symptoms. Runners who develop frequent recurrent attacks should consult a dermatologist or skin specialist for further advice. Diagnosis can be confirmed by analysis of blister fluid.

The other pattern of herpes simplex virus infection may involve any part of the body. This infection is contagious, being transmitted either sexually or by close body contact and can also be transmitted by contaminated clothing. It causes skin lesions or painful mouth blisters. Team epidemics may develop among athletes such as wrestlers who are involved in close physical contact. It also affects track men who share towels, running equipment or drinking cups. The blister is identical to the other type of herpes infection, and similarly, there is no specific treatment. Avoid it by careful hygiene in the locker room and on the track.

Please remember that infections of the feet and skin are usually due to poorly fitting shoes or sloppy personal hygiene. Once again, be smart. Use only clean equipment; use slippers or clogs in the locker room; don't share towels or drinking cups; keep the feet and groin dry and powdered; cover locker-room benches with towels; use cotton underpants under jock straps to prevent recurrent jock itch. If small lesions do develop, prompt attention will minimize the problem and prevent serious disability from infection.

FOOT VIRUSES (WARTS AND MOLLUSCUM CONTAGIOSUM)

Cause: Warts are viral infections of the skin. They are transmitted by personal contact and frequently infect runners' feet when they walk barefoot in the locker room or shower. Molluscum contagiosum is also a viral infection of the skin that is spread by contaminated towels, dirty floors and personal contact. All parts of the skin are susceptible.

Symptoms and Diagnosis: Warts are usually painless growths on the skin. Plantar warts, which are an exception, are quite painful. They grow in pressure spots such as the metatarsal area of the sole of the foot, and are frequently surrounded by heavy callus growth. Pressure from walking and running causes them to spread beneath the skin.

Molluscum contagiosum appears as pearly growths with indented centers. They are painless and contagious and may appear in clusters. When squeezed, thick white material is obtained.

Comments and Treatment: Runners may self-treat warts with 10% salicylic acid, 3% formaldehyde solution, or silver nitrate. Be careful, however, not to overtreat and burn the skin, causing scars. For this reason many trainers prefer tape impregnated with salicylic acid which is safer to use. Large warts must be removed with liquid nitrogen freezing or surgical dissection.

Plantar warts are best treated by a doctor or podiatrist because improper treatment may lead to tender scar tissue on the sole of the foot. You may get temporary relief of pain by placing a horseshoe-shaped piece of moleskin or chiropodist felt around a plantar wart (Figure 12-2). Needless to say, this disease is a runner's curse.

Molluscum contagiosum is treated with silver nitrate, liquid nitrogen or surgical removal.

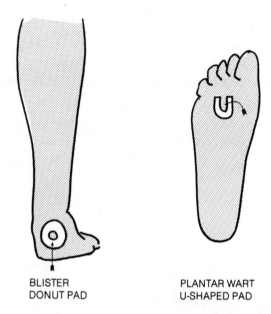

BLISTER   PLANTAR WART
DONUT PAD   U-SHAPED PAD

An adhesive felt donut placed on the skin adjacent to a blister prevents friction on the irritated site. A U-shaped or horseshoe pad relieves pressure on a plantar wart.

Figure 12-2. BLISTER AND PLANTAR WART TREATMENT

ALLERGIC DERMATITIS AND POISON IVY (SKIN ALLERGY)

Cause: A runner may become allergic to dye in shoes or socks, leather, adhesive tape, liniment, rubber or glue in shoes, elastic knee supports, elastic bands of shorts, or lime and chalk from the track. These materials mix with sweat, leading to itchy red skin lesions similar to poison ivy. If you run in the woods or in grassy areas near the track, you may indeed develop poison ivy. Allergic dermatitis has nothing to do with hygiene. It is strictly an allergy and just a matter of bad luck.

Symptoms and Diagnosis: Allergic dermatitis is an itchy red rash with occasional blisters, scales or crusts. The rash typically develops on skin usually covered by shoes or clothes. Common sites include the waist at the site of elastic bands in running shorts, the mid-back at the site of a metal bra clasp, knees wrapped with elastic supports, or skin under adhesive tape. If you don't wear socks, your feet can react to dyes, glues and shoe leather. Rashes on exposed skin suggest poison ivy.

Allergic dermatitis is a symmetrical rash. For example, it is equally severe on both feet, as opposed to infection which is usually worse on one side or the other. When in doubt a simple patch test can be performed. Place a small piece of the suspect material (leather, elastic, and so on) under adhesive tape on the lower back for 2 days. You will see an allergic rash when the tape is removed. Occasionally an allergist or dermatologist is needed to sort out difficult cases.

Most people recognize poison ivy. Remember that it requires only momentary contact with the leaves or vines of the plant, and thus you are frequently unaware of exposure.

Comments and Treatment: The obvious treatment of allergic dermatitis is to avoid the culprit material once it is identified. Fortunately, there are enough products on the market so the runner can obtain a nonallergenic substitute. Some people are very sensitive to poison ivy and must avoid all wooded and grassy areas. Long socks or sweat pants may be necessary for cross-country runners.

Poison ivy and allergic dermatitis are treated in similar ways. Severe cases are treated with warm water soaks. Cover rash with clean washcloth or bedsheet soaked in lukewarm tap water for about 15 minutes every few hours. Calamine lotion is soothing. Relieve itching with antihistamine pills (Atarax) and by washing with soap and very hot water. Very severe cases may require cortisone cream or pills. Allergy shots for poison ivy are controversial, and most experts don't think they help.

It may be impossible to remove poison ivy oil from clothing even with repeated washing, so discard contaminated garments.

HIVES OR URTICARIA

Cause: Hives are usually a sign of food allergy. But they may also be caused by physical agents that runners are frequently exposed to, such as:

Solar urticaria. Certain wavelengths of sunlight cause susceptible people to develop hives. This problem usually runs in fam-
ilies, but the exact mechanism is not clear.

Heat-induced or cholinergic urticaria. Runners are particularly prone to these disabling hives which occur when nerves in
the skin are stimulated by exercise in hot, humid environments.
Susceptible people first notice this tendency during childhood,
but it is usually a lifelong problem.

Cold urticaria. Probably the most common of runners' hives,
these appear on parts of the body exposed to low temperatures
such as the hands and legs. This problem usually develops suddenly in an otherwise healthy individual, and fortunately, it
tends to disappear after a year or two.

Symptoms and Diagnosis: Hives may be mildly uncomfortable
or completely disabling; most cases usually cause extreme itching. Very severe reactions can even lead to swelling of the mouth
and difficulty in breathing. Solar urticaria develops on parts of
the skin exposed to the sun. Heat-induced urticaria usually covers a large part of the body. Cold urticaria may cause very uncomfortable itching of the hands and wrists during cold weather.

The appearance of hives varies considerably. Lesions range in
size from several inches in diameter to smaller than the size of a
dime. Skin may be normal color, or large red welts may be present. In some instances, itching may be the only clue. Hives can
be easily distinguished from infections of the skin or contact
dermatitis by their duration. These latter rashes usually last several days, while hives disappear in a matter of hours.

Comments and Treatment: Because of increased exposure to sun,
heat, sweat and cold, runners develop hives more frequently
than other people. Food allergy, however, is still the most common cause of hives. When only one or two attacks occur, food is
more likely than physical factors.

Solar urticaria can be prevented with sunscreen creams. Attacks of heat urticaria may be minimized with antihistamines
(Atarax). Some people, however, are very sensitive to this problem and should avoid competitive running in hot, humid
weather. Avoid cold urticaria by wearing gloves and other cloth-

ing to cover exposed skin. Antihistamines will also minimize these attacks.

PRICKLY HEAT

Cause: Prickly heat or miliaria is due to obstruction of sweat pores during hot, humid weather. Some people are prone to this problem.

Symptoms and Diagnosis: Symptoms of prickly heat are quite characteristic and may be extremely uncomfortable. Itching, burning or stinging of the skin occurs as small red bumps or blisters suddenly develop during exercise in hot, humid weather. Repeated attacks are common. Careful examination of skin with a magnifying glass will show that the rash surrounds sweat pores and not hair follicles.

Comments and Treatment: Unfortunately, there is no specific treatment for prickly heat, but the condition is seldom severe enough to cause major problems. Well-ventilated clothing will help minimize accumulation of sweat on the skin. To avoid uncomfortable attacks on hot, humid days, shorten workouts.

CHAFING

Cause: Superficial irritation of the epidermis or outer layer of the skin is called chafing. This is caused by friction from contact with another surface such as tight-fitting clothing, running shoes or another area of body skin. Some runners develop chafing on the inner thighs, the scrotum, under the arms, over the nipples and where elastic such as pants bands and bra straps touch skin.

Symptoms and Diagnosis: Chafing causes local pain, tenderness and redness of the skin at areas of friction. Sometimes it must be differentiated from a hot spot described later. Chafing is more superficial and usually does not lead to the development of a blister.

Comments and Treatment: Eliminate potential causes such as tight-fitting shoes, running shorts or shirts to prevent chafing.

Long distance runners are frequently troubled by chafing in the groin, the inner thighs and the nipples, which can often be prevented or relieved by liberal administration of petroleum jelly. In other instances, such as severe nipple chafing, Band-Aids must be used to protect the irritated surfaces.

BLISTERS

Cause: Prolonged friction can cause abnormal fluid accumulation between the skin's inner and outer layers (Figure 12-2). These blisters frequently occur when a runner uses new shoes, when running on hot surfaces, when socks become wrinkled or during a very long race such as a marathon. Additional friction may cause bleeding into the blister from a rupture of small blood vessels, leading to a "blood blister."

Symptoms and Diagnosis: Usually a local "hot spot" of irritation will appear before a blister develops. Sometimes runners will note discomfort or mild pain when a hot spot or blister begins. At other times, however, especially during competition, a runner may completely block out blister pain until the race is over. Blisters at the tip of the toenail may extend under the toenail and cause bleeding and extreme pain. Large blisters can be completely disabling.

Comments and Treatment: Blisters can frequently be avoided. New shoes should be broken in slowly. Experienced runners rotate training shoes and never race or run long distances in new shoes. Some runners find that a thin pair of socks worn under heavier cotton or wool athletic socks will prevent blisters. Others who prefer running without socks rub petroleum jelly or lanolin on their feet and wear snug-fitting shoes. Cut toenails short to prevent friction from socks or tips of shoes.

When a hot spot develops, cover it with petroleum jelly and adhesive tape or moleskin.

Blisters should not be opened routinely unless there is severe pain or infection. Instead, cover them with petroleum jelly and adhesive tape or moleskin wrapped completely around the toe or foot. Packaged Band-Aids usually do not adhere well to the foot. A blister on the heel can be protected with a donut-shaped

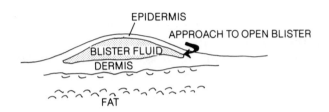

Chronic friction causes tissue injury and accumulation of fluid between the epidermis and dermis.

Figure 12-3.   ANATOMY OF A BLISTER

piece of felt taped in place around the margin of the blister (Figure 12-3).

When a blister causes considerable pain or when it is filled with pus, it should be opened. First wash the skin with plain soap and water. Then swab the site with 70% alcohol or iodine. Use a sterile razor blade or scissor to cut open the blister around the rim, wide enough to allow adequate drainage. Do not remove the skin over the blister. Once the fluid is drained, cover the blister with antibiotic ointment (Neosporin), sterile gauze and adhesive tape. Within 48 hours most blisters are dry enough to allow exposure to open air. With repeated friction, callus will develop at the site of a blister.

A blister may lead to bacterial infection. Pain or redness that lasts for more than 2 days or the presence of pus indicates infection. Infected blisters should be opened. Persistent infection must be treated by a doctor.

CALLUSES

Cause: Repeated episodes of long-standing, intermittent or continuous friction or pressure on the skin will cause thickening of the outer layer. Because these calluses are a natural protective reaction that toughens the skin, some degree of callus over pressure sites is desirable. Calluses may also develop because of ill-fitting shoes or deformities of the bony structure of the foot. Frequent sites of callus formation are the side of the fifth toe; the tips of the second, third and fourth toes; the heel; and the sole beneath the metatarsal heads.

Symptoms and Diagnosis: Calluses are usually painless. Occasionally, the involved skin is numb. When they become too thick they may pull on surrounding skin, causing pain and in some cases, blisters. Color varies from light yellow to brown. Close examination will reveal that normal epidermal ridges or "fingerprint" lines are visible.

Comments and Treatment: Each sport has characteristic callus formation described by eponyms such as bowler's thumb, jockey's buttocks, tennis or golfer's palm, and writer's finger. However, callus growth must be controlled because skin will lose its elasticity when a callus becomes too thick. Therefore, remove excess callus with a file or sandpaper. In addition, frequent application of petroleum jelly will keep the callus soft and help maintain elasticity. Thick painful calluses should be treated by a podiatrist.

CORNS

Cause: A corn can develop from prolonged or intermittent pressure on skin lying over a bony prominence. These very hard growths extend deeper into the skin than a callus. They are frequently associated with bony abnormalities of the feet or ill-fitting shoes.

Symptoms and Diagnosis: Corns are frequently painful and tender and can be distinguished from calluses by their hardness and the absence of epidermal ridges or fingerprint lines.

Comments and Treatment: Sometimes corns can be dissolved with commercial corn remover solutions or salicylic acid-impregnated tape. Surgical excision might be necessary for resistant cases. To relieve pressure over a corn, tape donut-shaped moleskin or a felt pad around the periphery.

Unfortunately, many corns will recur unless the underlying problem is corrected. Corns on the top of the second, third, or fourth toes indicate that running shoes are too tight. Flatfeet can cause corns beneath the metatarsal heads. Corns of the large toe are frequently associated with malalignment of the first metatarsal joint. Many of these problems can be solved with orthotics carefully designed by a podiatrist specializing in runners' problems. Extreme cases may require surgery to correct the bony deformity. This can best be performed by an orthopedic surgeon.

RAYNAUD'S DISEASE (DEAD FINGERS)

Cause: Many people suffer from Raynaud's disease, decreased blood flow to the hands during exposure to cold weather. The usual cause is spasm of arteries that supply blood to the fingers. While some cases are associated with serious diseases, the vast majority occur in otherwise healthy people. Fingers of both hands are usually involved. Women are more susceptible than men, and smoking aggravates the disease.

Symptoms and Diagnosis: The tips of the fingers will turn white or blue when exposed to cold or, in some cases, only mildly cool temperatures. Intense redness will occur when the fingers are rewarmed. Numbness, tingling and pain (sometimes severe) are usually present. Attacks may last from several minutes to an hour. The degree of sensitivity varies to the extent that some people experience Raynaud's disease when they wash their hands with cold water, while others have problems only under very cold environmental conditions. Occasionally, the toes will also be involved. When Raynaud's disease is long-standing, small areas of superficial gangrene may be noted.

Comments and Treatment: Cold weather runners commonly experience Raynaud's disease. If symptoms develop, consult a physician in order to exclude serious illnesses sometimes associated with this disorder. If none is found, minimize the symptoms by wearing gloves or mittens and thermal liners to help protect fingers from the cold. No specific medication has proven uniformly effective for the treatment of Raynaud's disease. But drugs that block blood vessel nerves are occasionally successful. Discuss these agents with a doctor if the problem becomes severe.

13

Infections

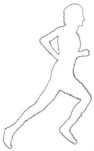

Runners are not immune from infections. On the contrary, many microorganisms take advantage of runners' health habits, causing a variety of problems. Despite antibiotics, infections should never be taken lightly. Yet many well-trained runners try to ignore minor infections and fevers. These dreamers are usually jolted back to reality by determined microorganisms that have no respect for trained bodies.

Infections are caused by viruses, bacteria and fungi, which enter the body through breaks in the skin, by oral ingestion and by inhalation of contaminated water droplets in the air. Healthy intact skin, stomach acid that destroys many bacteria, and antibody proteins that kill microorganisms in the airways are the body's first-line defenses against infection. Once infection begins, white blood cells and blood antibodies combine to kill the invaders and halt their spread. Fever, local redness, swelling and tenderness are signs of the body's normal inflammatory reaction to infection. Pus is a mixture of bacteria, white blood cells and tissue debris, the by-product of infection and inflammation.

Since there is no specific treatment for most viral infections, it is fortunate that they are usually mild and self-limited. On the other hand, bacterial and fungal infections frequently require antibiotics to speed recovery.

Runners are at risk from infections in several ways. Some viral diseases such as myocarditis (heart infection), influenza and polio are worsened by exercise. Running can prolong these infectious diseases and even cause fatality. Resistance to infections such as the common cold is often lowered during periods of hard training. Why and how this happens is unclear. Runners are also more frequently exposed to infections. For example, scratches of the skin can lead to tetanus or streptoccal infection. Other infections are contracted by running in wooded areas infested with disease-carrying insects such as ticks and mosquitos.

While most runners are certainly very healthy, they have no greater protection against infection than do nonrunners. But one of the greatest problems runners face is the "superman complex." We sometimes think ourselves indestructible and foolishly continue to train with minor colds, viral infections and fevers. As a result, we push ourselves too far and aggravate the condition. *Running with fever is stupid, dangerous and occasionally fatal.* Running with bacterial skin infections of the foot can spread infection and even drive it into the bloodstream. (Skin infections are discussed in Chapter 12.)

Common Cold

Cause: There are hundreds of different strains of viruses that cause the common cold. Infection is transmitted by close personal contact and not from exposure to cold temperatures. But wet, cold climates do increase susceptibility to cold viruses.

Symptoms and Diagnosis: Runny nose, sneezing, head congestion, low-grade fever, muscle aches and mild sore throat are all common cold symptoms. High fever, thick discolored sputum or nasal discharge, intense cough and excessive fatigue all suggest more serious infections such as sinusitis (bacterial infection of the sinuses), strep throat and pneumonia.

Comments and Treatment: Antihistamines, drugstore cold remedies and nasal sprays minimize head congestion. Aspirin relieves fever, headache and muscle pain. Running can prolong cold symptoms and even precipitate secondary bacterial infection such as sinusitis and bronchitis. It is reasonable to continue light running with a mild cold, but curtail hard workouts. If symptoms worsen or do not improve in 48 hours, stop running altogether and rest for a few days to regain strength. Continued training will only tear down the body and prolong the illness.

Sore Throat

Cause: Viral infections, streptococcus bacteria, infectious mononucleosis and allergies can all cause sore throat. Each runner must decide whether or not these common diseases are severe enough to interfere with training and competitive running.

Symptoms and Diagnosis: Each of the above diseases can produce sore throat symptoms that range from mild scratchy throat to extreme pain and difficulty in swallowing. High fever and tender glands in the neck suggest streptococcal infection. A throat culture for streptococcus should be done within the first 2 days of illness. This disease usually subsides within a few days. Mononucleosis, which is diagnosed from a blood smear and a special mono-spot test performed with a blood sample, often causes swollen glands, mild jaundice and lingering fatigue. Other viral infections usually clear in 2 days. Itchy eyes and sneezing often accompany allergic sore throat. Allergic people develop these symptoms after they eat certain foods or inhale dust and pollens. Frequent episodes are usual.

Comments and Treatment: Viral sore throat should be treated with aspirin and rest and usually improves within 2 days. A simple viral sore throat is not aggravated by running.

There is danger of heart damage from rheumatic fever following streptococcal sore throat (see Chapter 15). Youngsters are especially susceptible to this complication. For this reason, strep throat should always be treated with penicillin. Young runners (under twenty) and runners with a past history of rheumatic fever should not train hard for at least 2 weeks after a strep throat.

Mononucleosis may last for several weeks. Complete cessation of running is absolutely necessary during the acute phase, for not only can running prolong recovery, but there is also a danger of a ruptured spleen from vigorous exercise. When appetite improves, fatigue disappears and fever is completely gone, gradual resumption of running is safe. However, infectious mononucleosis does occasionally relapse, in which case it should be treated by a physician. Fortunately you almost never get infectious mono more than once.

Allergic sore throat improves with antihistamines and avoidance of allergenic substances.

Influenza

Cause: Influenza virus is transmitted from person to person by coughing and sneezing. It infects both the upper and lower respiratory tracts and spreads to the bloodstream and the rest of the body. Most cases are self-limited. Older people, pregnant women and individuals with chronic disease can develop complications. Each year new types of viruses spread across the country, causing outbreaks and epidemics during the winter months.

Symptoms and Diagnosis: Influenza causes sudden chills, high fever, headache, severe muscle aches, cough, sore throat, diarrhea and occasional vomiting. Symptoms usually occur in winter months during local epidemics. A blood test confirms diagnosis, but it takes weeks to obtain positive results.

Comments and Treatment: Aspirin and fluids help control symptoms and absolute rest is mandatory. Never run with influenza. This particular infection is almost certainly aggravated by vigorous exercise and may cause infection of the heart (see below). Symptoms usually improve in 3 or 4 days and you can safely resume running 2 days after fever disappears. Postpone hard workouts for at least a week.

Myocarditis (infection of the heart)

Cause: Influenza and Coxsackie viruses are the most common cause of myocarditis. These viruses directly infect the heart muscle, causing local inflammation and destruction of muscle fibers. Weakened cardiac muscle can lead to heart failure.

Symptoms and Diagnosis: Myocarditis usually follows influenza or coldlike illnesses. Chest pain, shortness of breath while resting or running, extreme fatigue, ankle swelling, skipped heart beats and fever suggest myocarditis.

It is a very serious disease and should be evaluated by a physician or a cardiologist (heart specialist). Electrocardiogram, chest X ray and ultrasound study of the heart will probably all be performed.

Comments and Treatment: Hospitalization and several weeks of strict bedrest are necessary in treating myocarditis. Recovery takes months and permanent heart damage is common. While myocarditis is fortunately relatively rare, every year a few runners die suddenly from it. This is a major reason that experts caution against running with any fever, influenza or a severe cold. Exercise during myocarditis infection can definitely be fatal, and we strongly recommend that a runner who develops myocarditis be treated by a cardiologist.

Hepatitis

Cause: Hepatitis is a viral infection of the liver produced by several different types of viruses. Runners have an increased risk of serum hepatitis (hepatitis type B) and infectious hepatitis (hepatitis type A).

Serum hepatitis is transmitted by a small amount of infected blood that enters the body through a scratch or skin abrasion. Several years ago there was a large outbreak of hepatitis B among Swedish long distance runners. These infected runners scratched their legs in the underbrush, leaving small drops of blood containing hepatitis virus. Other competitors then scratched themselves on the same branches and acquired infection. After competition they bathed in communal pools that were also probably contaminated with virus.

Infectious hepatitis type A is transmitted by oral ingestion of hepatitis A virus. Drinking water contaminated with sewage is a common source and often consumed by runners at wells or streams in the woods or at overcrowded running events with poor sanitation.

Symptoms and Diagnosis: Loss of appetite, fatigue, dark urine, yellow eyes and skin, vomiting, joint pain, and itchy skin are all symptoms of hepatitis. They develop about 30 days after ingestion of hepatitis A and about 90 days after exposure to hepatitis B.

Suspected cases should be brought to the attention of a doctor who will perform a blood test to evaluate liver damage and to detect the virus in the blood.

Comments and Treatment: There is no specific treatment for viral hepatitis. Recovery almost always occurs, but it usually takes 2–6 weeks. While mild exercise will not aggravate most cases, it is still uncertain what effect hard training will have. It is best to stop running until liver function improves (this is determined by periodic blood tests), and once recovery begins, resume light running. But if relapse of liver disease occurs, stop all running for at least 2 additional weeks.

The severe outbreak among the Swedish runners was controlled by prohibiting running with bare legs. When this ban was suspended, the hepatitis epidemic recurred.

One year hepatitis A from a contaminated water fountain infected most of the Holy Cross football team members, resulting in cancellation of the entire season. A Connecticut team was decimated by hepatitis B that contaminated shared shaving razors.

When outbreaks of hepatitis affect a track team, a doctor should be consulted to help find the source of the infection. Gammaglobulin will minimize symptoms of those exposed, and this treatment should be considered for the teammates of infected runners.

A smart runner can protect himself from these dangers by not drinking from streams or wells. Bring your own water or drink bottled liquid at races where sanitation is questionable. Avoid shared equipment whenever possible.

Food Poisoning

Cause: Salmonella, staphylococcus, clostridium and other bacteria contaminate food such as pastry, chicken, seafood and powdered milk. When food is not prepared under sanitary conditions or is not refrigerated, bacteria grow and produce poisons called toxins. Unsuspecting people who eat this food will suffer extreme gastrointestinal upset, and when several people who shared a meal develop vomiting or diarrhea, food poisoning is probable.

Symptoms and Diagnosis: Diarrhea, vomiting and occasional fever develop from 1–48 hours after eating contaminated food. Symptoms can be completely disabling and dehydration may develop. Bacteria and toxins may be isolated from leftover food or from a patient's stool and blood.

Comments and Treatment: Food poisoning is a danger to runners who eat at county fairs and local festivals associated with road-racing events. Tempting home-cooked food at these fairs is sometimes prepared under unsanitary conditions or is not refrigerated. A high degree of caution against eating home-cooked foods at these events will prevent considerable discomfort. Contaminated food may look and taste completely normal.

Most cases improve with no special treatment. Severe illness may require hospitalization and intravenous fluids for dehydration. In general, avoid antibiotics and antidiarrheal drugs because they may actually prolong the illness. Since there is considerable fluid and salt loss from diarrhea and vomiting, resume running slowly to allow replenishment of body fluids and electrolytes. Postpone any long runs, especially in hot weather, for at least a week after recovery from this illness.

Tetanus

Cause: Tetanus is a serious infection caused by a bacteria called Clostridium tetani which survives for years as a dry spore in soil. When a small cut or puncture wound of the skin is contaminated by the spores, bacteria begin to grow and cause a local infection. These bacteria produce a very potent poison called a toxin which enters the bloodstream and damages the brain and nervous system. Infected individuals develop convulsions, muscle spasm and inability to open the mouth (lockjaw). Death from suffocation frequently occurs.

Symptoms and Diagnosis: Tetanus infection can develop in a very minor skin injury. The symptoms of this local infection are often so minimal that they are unrecognized until signs of nervous system disease occur.

Comments and Treatment: People with tetanus are gravely ill and need immediate medical care. Individuals who develop convulsions or severe muscle spasm require emergency hospital care. Fortunately tetanus can be prevented. Immunization is a simple injection that affords the body immunity to tetanus toxin for at least ten years. Most people are immunized during childhood; men are always inoculated when inducted into the armed services. Unfortunately not everyone in this country receives immunization, and each year there are still several hundred tetanus cases. We recommend that you receive booster immunizations every ten years in order to maintain resistance. In most cases this is adequate protection, although when you receive a puncture wound or laceration, you are frequently given a tetanus booster shot. Hypothetically, this helps reinforce the body's immunity.

Runners have a high risk of tetanus since minor cuts and abrasions of their legs and feet are common. All runners would be wise to check their immunization schedule to make sure that they have had a tetanus booster within the last ten years.

Tick Fevers and Tick Paralysis

Cause: Wooded areas are usually infested with ticks that may cling to the socks and clothing of runners in the woods. While tick bites may not be noticed, ticks cause at least three different diseases in the United States: Rocky Mountain spotted fever caused by a viruslike microorganism; Colorado tick fever caused by a virus; tick paralysis caused by a poison excreted by the tick.

Symptoms and Diagnosis: Rocky Mountain spotted fever causes a rash and fever. This disease is serious and occasionally fatal. Colorado tick fever causes a mild fever that lasts about a week. Infected people frequently cannot recall a tick bite. Tick paralysis usually affects children, resulting in paralysis and occasional death. In contrast to tick fevers, this disease occurs while the insect is still imbedded in the skin.

Comments and Treatment: In 1977 there were more than 1,000 cases of tick fever, and the problem is increasing yearly. Rocky Mountain spotted fever occurs throughout most of the central and eastern United States. Colorado tick fever occurs in the western states. Both illnesses are seasonal with peaks in the spring and summer. Cross-country runners and others who run in the woods are most likely to become infected after runs. These individuals should check their bodies and clothing for ticks. In addition, pet dogs frequently bring ticks into the home. Fatalities from Rocky Mountain spotted fever and tick paralysis can occur if the diagnosis is not made during the early stages of the disease. When an unexplained fever occurs, usually 2 days to 2 weeks after a tick bite or exposure to ticks, bring it to the attention of a doctor. Blood tests are available to diagnose Rocky Mountain spotted fever and Colorado tick fever. Rocky Mountain spotted fever is treated with antibiotics (chloramphenicol and tetracycline), but there is no specific treatment for Colorado tick fever. A child who runs or plays in the woods and develops paralysis should be carefully examined for ticks. When the insect is removed, prompt recovery occurs.

Lice

Runners may develop an infection with different varieties of lice that attack man. These include the head louse, body louse and the pubic or crab louse. These insects attach to body hairs and feed on human blood. Extreme itching, skin infection and more serious diseases can be transmitted by body lice. Lice are spread by close personal contact and from bedding and toilet seats, as well as through stacked gym towels, team uniforms, locker room floors and benches, making runners and other athletes particularly susceptible. This infection may result from either poor personal hygiene or from contamination of shared equipment or improperly stored towels and uniforms. If a runner develops lice, he should completely bathe his body with 1% lindane (Kwell shampoo). All clothing and bedding should be thoroughly cleaned.

14

The Respiratory System

Problems of the airways and lungs are often neglected by runners. These marvelous organs filter and humidify polluted air, presenting pure oxygen to the body in exchange for waste products. Many runners are plagued by sneezing, coughing, allergies and sinus problems while others are unaware that they suffer from "runners' asthma," a subtle form of disease that can impede running performance without causing symptoms.

BASIC STRUCTURE AND FUNCTION

When we breathe air through the nose and mouth, it travels to the lungs via a main passageway called the trachea. In the chest, the airways branch into smaller and smaller tubes, finally ending in thin saclike membranes of lung tissue surrounded by small capillary blood vessels. The respiratory system can be divided into the upper airway, which includes the nose, mouth, sinuses and trachea; and the lower airway, which includes branching air passages called bronchi and lung tissue (Figure 14-1).

The main function of the upper airway is to process air before

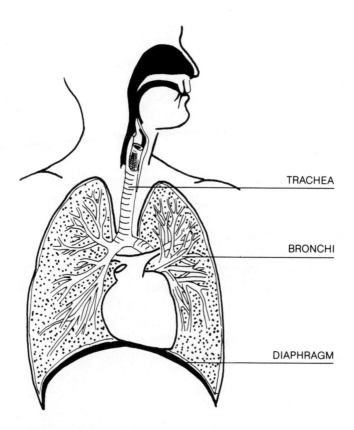

Air travels through the trachea into the branching bronchi which end in the terminal airway (Figure 14-3). The diaphragm and intercostal muscles between the ribs act as a bellows to move air in and out of the lungs.

Figure 14-1.   THE RESPIRATORY SYSTEM

it reaches the lung. At rest, most of the air we breathe passes through the nasal passages where it undergoes air filtration, humidification and temperature regulation. Air is filtered when small dust particles are trapped in a thick blanket of mucus lining the nasal passages. Water vapor is added to inspired air to achieve a relative humidity of 85–90 percent by the time it reaches the trachea. In addition, the nose has a remarkable ability to heat inhaled air regardless of outside temperatures so that it is only 1–2° C above or below body temperature when it reaches the pharynx (throat). The sinuses are cavities in the bony skull which are lined with mucous membranes similar to that in the nose and mouth. There are frontal sinuses over the eyebrows and maxillary and sphenoid sinuses under the eyes (Figure 14-2). While their exact function is unknown, they probably play a role in the humidification and heating of inhaled air. The trachea, or main airway, is a long tube surrounded by supporting rings of cartilage and covered with a mucous membrane that helps complete the process of heating, humidification, and air filtration.

The lower respiratory tract consists of a series of airways that branch into smaller and smaller units, finally ending in thin air/gas exchange sac units called alveoli. The medium-sized airways are surrounded by smooth muscle which contracts and relaxes to change the airways diameter. At the alveoli (Figure 14-3), oxygen diffuses from the lungs across a thin membrane into small capillary blood vessels, while carbon dioxide from the body's metabolic processes travels in the opposite direction. This diffusion process occurs very rapidly. When oxygen reaches the bloodstream, it is carried by hemoglobin protein in red blood cells. At rest, blood is maximally saturated with oxy-

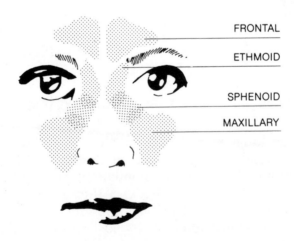

FRONTAL

ETHMOID

SPHENOID

MAXILLARY

Holes in the bony skull are called sinuses. Allergies and infections often cause inflammation of these structures (sinusitis).

Figure 14-2. SINUSES

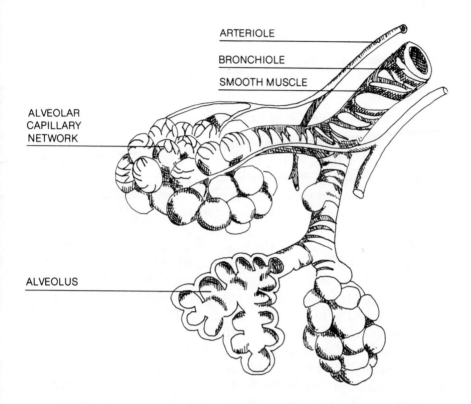

ARTERIOLE

BRONCHIOLE

SMOOTH MUSCLE

ALVEOLAR
CAPILLARY
NETWORK

ALVEOLUS

Inspired air reaches the alveolus through the bronchioles, the smallest of the branching air tubes. The alveolus is the air exchange unit where oxygen crosses a thin membrane to enter the rich capillary network of the bloodstream, and carbon dioxide travels in the opposite direction as it leaves the body. The smooth muscle that surrounds the bronchiole can constrict the airway, causing resistance to air flow and asthma.

Figure 14-3.   TERMINAL AIRWAY

gen. The body cannot store oxygen; therefore, there is no benefit from breathing pure oxygen before a race.

The lungs function like a bellows moving air in and out by expanding and contracting. This movement is accomplished by intercostal muscles between the ribs, by the muscular diaphragm, and by the abdominal muscles. When we inhale, the lungs expand causing a negative pressure which draws air into the lungs. When we exhale, lung tissue contracts forcing air out of the lungs.

The amount of air entering the lungs with each breath is called the tidal volume and is approximately 500 milliliters at rest. Most people breathe about twelve times a minute at rest resulting in a resting ventilatory rate of approximately 6 liters per minute.

Respiratory Changes with Exercise

During exercise mouth breathing is necessary to accommodate the increased volume of inhaled air. As a result, much of this air bypasses the nasal passages, thereby losing the benefits of filtration, humidification and temperature regulation. Thus, air reaching the lungs during heavy exercise is often drier and cooler than air inhaled at rest.

Tidal volume increases during exercise to reach a *maximum inspiratory capacity* of approximately 3½ liters. The number of breaths per minute also increase to about 40 per minute. The amount of air inhaled per minute during maximum exercise is called the *maximum breathing capacity*. Elite athletes attain values between 150–200 liters per minute.

The body uses more oxygen during exercise. However, oxygen diffuses across the pulmonary capillaries so fast that there is no difficulty resupplying blood with enough oxygen to saturate the red blood cells' carrying capacity. Likewise, the amount of carbon dioxide brought to the lungs from exercising muscle is increased. But this gas can also quickly diffuse out of the blood into the exhaled air so that it does not build up in the body.

Training the Respiratory Stystem

The upper airway undergoes no specific adaptations to training. In addition, there is no change in the number of air sacs or the capillary network of the lungs. But trained distance runners do have a slight increase in the lungs' inspiratory capacity and total lung volume. More important, the maximum breathing capacity is increased and can be maintained for long periods of time. This probably results from increased endurance and strengthening of the respiratory muscles. As a result, elite distance runners can maintain volumes of 120–150 liters per minute during long races.

Another unique characteristic of some endurance runners appears to be inherited. There is a control center in the brain that signals the lungs to increase respiration when low oxygen or high carbon dioxide is detected in the blood. Some people are born with a relative insensitivity to these respiratory stimuli. As a result, they can tolerate much lower blood oxygen and higher carbon dioxide than can most individuals. Many good distance runners have this genetic advantage.

Diseases of the Upper Airways

Runners are plagued by a variety of symptoms involving the upper airways. While most of these diseases are relatively minor, they can interfere with performance and ruin running enjoyment. Problems include sneezing, coughing, hay fever and other allergies, stuffy or runny nose and sinus disease.

SNEEZING

Cause: Sneezing is a reflex mechanism caused by irritation of the mucous membranes of the nose. Irritation may result from air pollution, infections such as the common cold, allergic reactions, or from dryness of the mucous membranes. Other causes include vasomotor rhinitis (discussed in this chapter) and an inherited tendency to sneeze in bright light.

Symptoms and Diagnosis: Careful analysis of the circumstances surrounding bouts of sneezing will usually pinpoint the cause. A runner who suffers from sneezing in the spring or fall, especially in association with itchy eyes and a watery nose, should suspect an allergy. Sneezing produced by a cold usually clears within a week. Runners who train in dry climates or high altitudes may develop dryness, crusting or even shallow ulcers of the nasal mucous membranes. The sneezing reflex due to bright light usually causes sneezing bouts for the first few minutes of exposure to sunlight. This symptom then gradually disappears.

Comments and Treatment: Nasal sprays containing decongestants may prevent sneezing from air pollution, allergies and colds. Antihistamine pills are also helpful. Dry nose symptoms usually respond to moisture, and a simple remedy is application of a thin coat of petroleum jelly to the inside of the nose. More resistant cases may require humidified air. A runner who lives in a dry climate might benefit from a humidifier in the house or bedroom.

COUGHING

Cause: A cough is a reflex due to irritation of the upper airway or trachea. The most common causes are infections, allergies and air pollution. The cough reflex is a very important mechanism to protect the lower airway from foreign particles. The upper airway cannot completely filter all of the small particles from the air as it passes to the lungs. To keep the airways clear, substances such as pollens and dust must be continually removed from the lungs. These particles are trapped in thick mucus that lines the major airways. Particle-laden mucus travels up the airways to the top of the trachea where it is swallowed. Coughing facilitates this clearing process by pushing mucus out of the trachea.

Symptoms: Many runners who don't cough during daily runs will experience severe attacks during intense workouts and races. These symptoms result from dryness. The large volume of air inhaled during hard running is not humified. As a consequence, the mucus in the trachea dries, making it difficult to remove. Coughing episodes are merely the body's attempt to raise and clear dried mucus.

Comments and Treatment: Occasional coughing during running is a necessary and desirable mechanism that should not be of concern. If you are very sensitive to air pollution and dust, avoid dirt tracks, dusty trails and traffic-congested roads, and you might sometimes wear a paper mask to filter larger particles from the air.

Excessive coughing at rest or during light workouts suggests diseases such as infections or allergies. Sometimes a persistent cough defies analysis. Occasionally it is a sign of a serious disease such as a tumor of the airway or lungs. When a chronic cough persists, consult a doctor for complete evaluation.

HAY FEVER AND OTHER ALLERGIES

Cause: About 15 percent of adults develop allergies. These people are sensitive to certain foreign substances containing protein. Allergic symptoms are the result of the body's response to these allergenic proteins. Most often, plant pollen, house dust or animal dander comes in contact with the mucous membranes of the eyes or nose. The body reacts by liberating a chemical substance called histamine, which produces redness, congestion, and irritation of the mucous membranes. Symptoms such as itching, swelling of the nose and eyes and sneezing develop. In other cases, pollens may reach the lungs, causing an asthma attack.

In addition to pollens and other irritants in the air, allergic reactions can occur after eating various foods. The most common offenders include shellfish, alcoholic beverages, cheeses, dairy products, chocolate, spices, and various fruits, but essentially every type of food has caused allergic symptoms at some time. The tendency to develop allergic reactions is inherited. Most people who are exposed to pollens, dust, and other allergens for their whole life never develop symptoms, while others are allergic to numerous substances.

Symptoms and Diagnosis: Allergic symptoms usually begin within a few minutes of exposure to the allergenic substance, although food allergy reactions may be delayed for several hours. Allergy to tree, grass and ragweed pollens occurs during specific pollination seasons which vary from one geographic region of the country to another. Allergy to dust, molds, and animals produces year-round symptoms, which are usually worse in the winter when people spend more time indoors.

Individuals who note seasonal symptoms such as itchy eyes, sneezing, chronic "colds," scratchy throats, coughing, head congestion or wheezing may be suffering from an allergy. Family history of allergy is common. An allergist can determine if symptoms are allergic. He will take a careful history and perform skin tests with small samples of suspected material. These tests indicate which substances are responsible for allergic symptoms.

Comments and Treatment: Seasonal pollen allergy can be particularly bothersome to runners who spend many hours out-of-doors. Severe allergic symptoms can block air passageways, making breathing difficult. Excess mucus production can produce postnasal drip, resulting in coughing and gagging. Seasonal asthma sometimes occurs. Conversely, many runners report that their allergic symptoms clear during running. This improvement might be produced by adrenalin secreted into the blood during heavy exercise.

Fortunately, runners can do several things to minimize allergic symptoms. A person who awakens each day of the year with itchy eyes, sneezing, postnasal drip, and congested nose is probably allergic to dust, molds, the family pet or some other article in the home and should institute dust control measures in their home, particularly in the bedroom. Air filtration machines are also helpful.

Those runners whose symptoms are clearly limited to pollination seasons should focus their attention on those troublesome months, using nose sprays containing cortisone or adrenalinlike substances to shrink swollen mucous membranes. Antihistamine pills help itchy eyes, sinus congestion and sneezing.

If your symptoms interfere with running and other vital functions, consult an allergist. He might recommend desensitization shots. These injections contain very small amounts of the allergenic protein. Over a period of several months, your body gradually develops immunity to the offending substance. Allergy shots are often helpful but don't always work. Generally avoid cortisone for treatment of mild allergies because it has several adverse side effects.

VASOMOTOR RHINITIS

Cause: Some people possess unusually sensitive nasal membranes and develop symptoms such as sneezing and nasal congestion that resemble an allergy attack. Their symptoms, however, are not really allergic. These individuals are unduly sensitive to changes in the environment such as strong smells, sudden changes in temperature or humidity, cigarette smoke and other air pollutants. Even vigorous exercise such as running can cause these symptoms.

Symptoms and Diagnosis: As stated, the symptoms resemble allergic nasal congestion but usually without seasonal variation. Many people with allergies also suffer from vasomotor rhinitis.

An allergist can confirm a diagnosis of vasomotor rhinitis when allergy skin tests are negative and by microscopic examination of a smear of nasal mucus.

Comments and Treatment: Antihistamines and decongestant nose sprays often prevent vasomotor rhinitis. Take these medications about one-half hour before a workout.

SINUSITIS

Cause: Infection of the paranasal sinuses can be very disabling. These sinuses normally drain into the nose and throat through small channels. However, when allergy or viral infection cause swelling of mucous membranes, sinus passageways may be blocked. Mucus accumulation leads to increased pressure within the sinus cavities, causing pain and headache. Bacterial infection frequently develops, producing fever and fatigue. This condition is called acute sinusitis.

Some people suffer from chronic sinusitis. Their mucous membranes are thick and chronically inflamed, usually the result of long-standing allergies. Partial or intermittent blockage of sinus drainage occurs, producing congestion, headache and recurrent acute sinusitis.

Symptoms and Diagnosis: Attacks of acute sinusitis usually cause severe discomfort. In addition to headache and pain over the eyebrows or under the eyes, fever, chills and bloody or pussy discharge from the nose are often present. Chronic sinusitis can also cause chronic headaches, sinus pain or morning postnasal drip, runny nose or sputum production and fatigue. Sinus headache is aggravated by body movements that lower the head, such as toe-touching exercises.

Acute sinusitis can be diagnosed by examination and X ray of the sinuses. Runners with chronic headache and congestion may have chronic sinusitis which is often difficult to recognize. They should consult their family physician or an ear, nose and throat specialist. Examination of the internal mucous membranes will frequently reveal chronic changes.

Comments and Treatment: Acute sinusitis is a serious infection that requires antibiotics, antihistamines and occasional surgical drainage. Runners who develop acute sinusitis should eliminate or drastically curtail workouts until infection has subsided.

Runners who are plagued by sinus problems during running or hard workouts, may also be suffering from chronic sinusitis. The vigorous exercise of running causes partial drainage of congested sinuses into the nose and throat. Antihistamine pills and decongestant nose sprays frequently alleviate this problem. But it may take weeks for these medications to shrink swollen membranes and relieve congestion. Surgery may be necessary when the sinuses are severely inflamed. Since most cases of chronic sinusitis are due to allergies, a complete allergy evaluation is recommended.

Other runners often note sinus headache, particularly in the front region over the eyebrows, when exercising in cold, dry climates or during races or speed workouts. The exact mechanism of this problem is unclear. Some of these runners probably suffer from a form of vasomotor rhinitis, while others appear to be very sensitive to air that is not properly warmed and humidified. Using a paper mask or a scarf wrapped around the nose and mouth during cold weather runs can often bring relief. (Also see section on Effort Headache, Chapter 20).

RUNNERS' ASTHMA

Cause: The airways leading to the lungs are surrounded by smooth muscle. When these muscles contract, the passageways are narrowed, making it difficult to move air in and out of the lungs. This is an asthmatic attack. It may result from allergy, air

pollution, infection or inherited factors. Many people also develop asthma during exercise, and running causes asthma more
frequently than any other form of exercise.

A surprisingly large number of people are susceptible to runners' asthma. It occurs in approximately two-thirds of people
who have other types of asthma. In addition, a high percentage
of people with allergies such as hay fever or eczema develop
asthma when they run. Most surprising, up to 5 percent of people with no history of asthma or allergies will suffer from asthma
during running. This disease is most common among children
but can affect any age group. Symptoms occur most often during
the spring and fall when there are plant pollens in the air and
during cold or humid environmental conditions.

Symptoms and Diagnosis: A runner may experience coughing,
wheezing, shortness of breath, heaviness in the chest or unusual
fatigue within a few minutes after beginning to run. Many people note that these initial asthma symptoms slowly improve after
10 or 15 minutes of running. This is called the run through
phenomenon and is correlated with adaptive changes in the
lungs.

Lungs are obviously important to supply adequate oxygen for
running. Runners' asthma causes at least a 10 percent impairment of pulmonary function. Performance will certainly suffer.
If a runner suspects that he had runners' asthma, routine medical
examination alone is not adequate. He must also be examined
while running, and in some cases, air flow through the lungs
must be measured with a spirometer. We are convinced from
personal experience that many runners who suffer from this
problem are unaware that they have asthma. They complain of
tightness or heaviness in the chest and nagging cough or poor
performance during certain seasons of the year or during cold
weather running. A specialist in chest diseases may be needed
to diagnose these subtle cases.

Comments and Treatment: There are several medications now
available that prevent or alleviate runners' asthma. Most experts
agree that cromolyn sodium and beta 2 adrenergic stimulators
such as salbutamol work best. These agents are frequently com-

bined for maximum results. Take salbutamol pills an hour before exercise, combined with aerosolized salbutamol and cromolyn sodium immediately prior to competition. Other drugs such as theophylline, ephedrine, atropine and aerosolized beclomethasone are also useful. Although there is some concern about heartbeat irregularities associated with these medications, this complication is apparently rare. Over-the-counter preparations are not as effective. An asthmatic runner should see a chest specialist for best results. You can avoid cold weather asthma by wearing a loose-fitting paper mask or scarf wrapped around the nose and mouth during training runs.

Despite medications, some individuals with asthma are unable to run. Many turn to swimming for exercise and competition. Of all strenuous sports, swimming causes the least exercise-induced asthma. In fact, asthmatics have won gold medals in swimming at the last five Olympiads. Rules of international competition unfortunately consider use of adrenergic drugs doping. An American competitor was disqualified from the 1972 Olympic summer games and his gold medal was confiscated when this medication was detected in his urine. Therefore, serious competitors who use these medications should check with officials before a major race.

15

The Cardiovascular System

The limits of a runner's ability are closely linked to the capacity of his heart. Every aspiring competitive runner must therefore understand the cardiovascular system and its adaptations to training, and every runner—competitive or not —should understand the symbiotic relationship between the heart and running. Just as the heart helps a runner perform, the benefits of running help keep the heart healthy.

Basic Structure and Function

The heart is a muscular pump that propels blood through the body's arteries and veins. Blood is pumped from the left side of the heart through arteries that supply oxygen to body tissues (Figure 15-1). Veins carry oxygen-poor blood back from the body to the right side of the heart where it is pumped to the lungs. Oxygen from inhaled air crosses through small blood vessels (capillaries) in the lungs to replenish the blood oxygen concentration. Oxygen-rich blood then returns to the left side of the heart where the cycle begins again. The heart must work continually, day and night, and heart muscle requires an uninterrupted supply of its own oxygen-rich blood to continue contracting.

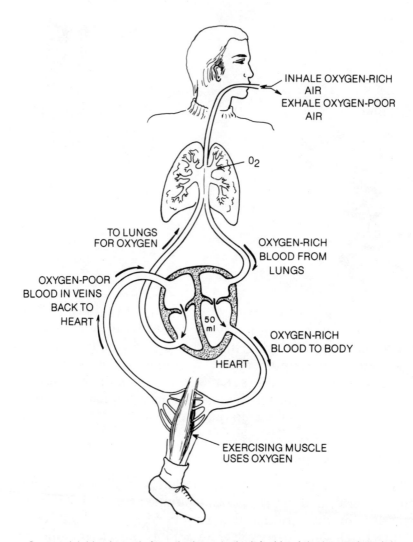

INHALE OXYGEN-RICH
AIR
EXHALE OXYGEN-POOR
AIR

O_2

TO LUNGS
FOR OXYGEN

OXYGEN-RICH
BLOOD FROM
LUNGS

OXYGEN-POOR
BLOOD IN VEINS
BACK TO
HEART

50
ml

OXYGEN-RICH
BLOOD TO BODY

HEART

EXERCISING MUSCLE
USES OXYGEN

Oxygen-rich blood travels from the lungs to the left side of the heart where it is pumped through arteries to the tissues of the body. In the capillaries, oxygen leaves the blood and enters the tissues as carbon dioxide, and other body wastes travel in the opposite direction. Oxygen-poor blood travels through veins to the lungs where it is replenished with oxygen.

Figure 15-1.   THE CARDIOVASCULAR SYSTEM

The two main coronary arteries travel through the heart muscle to supply oxygen for cardiac work (Figure 15-2).

In order for blood to be propelled effectively through the arteries, there must be adequate pressure within the cardiovascular system. Blood pressure is controlled by smooth muscles that line many of the body's arteries. Contraction or relaxation of these muscles will alter the internal diameter of the blood vessels, raising or lowering blood pressure in the whole system. When blood pressure increases, the heart must pump harder to propel blood, and when the pressure is too high, the heart is unable to pump effectively, resulting in heart failure.

The heart is composed of cardiac muscle which contracts

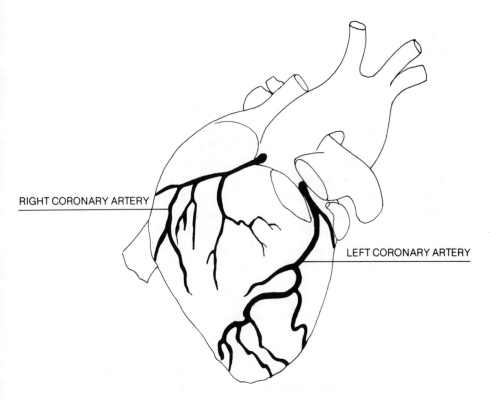

RIGHT CORONARY ARTERY

LEFT CORONARY ARTERY

The two coronary arteries arise at the root of the aorta and supply blood to the heart muscle.

Figure 15-2.   CORONARY ARTERIES

rhythmically. Each heartbeat represents a stroke of the pump, pushing blood through the blood vessels. Heart rate is controlled by nervous tone of the vagus and sympathetic nerves. Nervous signals pass through an electrical conducting system of the heart, synchronizing each contraction much like electricity passing along a flashing neon sign. At rest the heart beats between 40–80 times a minute. In addition to nervous control, a variety of chemical substances such as adrenalin and acidosis of the blood can affect heart rate. That amount of blood pumped with each heartbeat is called the *stroke volume* and is normally between 50–100 milliliters. The total amount of blood pumped by the heart per minute is called the *cardiac output* and is usually about 5 liters at rest.

Changes with Running

During exercise heart rate increases to a maximum of 150–200 beats per minute, and stroke volume also increases to 100–150 milliliters. As a result, during maximum exercise cardiac output can be increased about sixfold from 5 to 30 liters per minute.

Arteries can be visualized as pipes connected to the heart pump in a parallel arrangement (Figure 15-3). Blood flow is shunted from one part of the body to another by increasing the internal diameter of the vessels in one organ and narrowing the diameter in another. For example, after a meal blood flow is directed to the intestines and liver. Similarly, blood flow to muscle increases during exercise when the blood vessels that supply these muscles dilate and divert blood from the body's other organs. At rest skeletal muscle receives only 15 percent of the cardiac output. However, during maximum exercise such as running, blood flow to muscles may approach 85 percent of the total cardiac output. During exercise the heart must work harder to increase cardiac output. Therefore, the coronary arteries dilate to increase blood flow to the heart in order to keep up with increased oxygen demands of cardiac muscle. The end result of these physiologic changes is a twentyfold increase in oxygen supplied to exercising muscle.

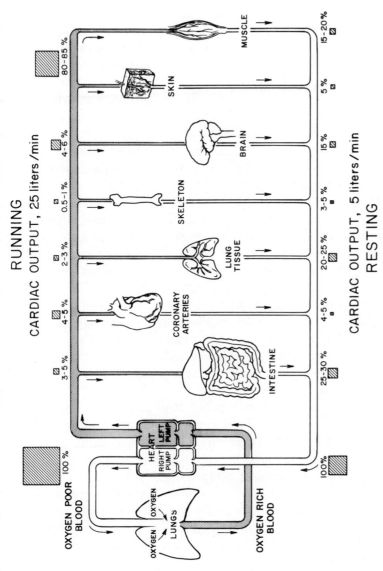

RUNNING
CARDIAC OUTPUT, 25 liters/min

80-85 %   4-6 %   0.5-1%   2-3 %   4-5 %   3-5 %

MUSCLE   SKIN   BRAIN   SKELETON   LUNG TISSUE   CORONARY ARTERIES   INTESTINE

15-20 %   5 %   15 %   3-5 %   20-25 %   4-5 %   25-30 %

RESTING
CARDIAC OUTPUT, 5 liters/min

HEART   RIGHT PUMP   LEFT PUMP

OXYGEN POOR BLOOD   100 %

100%

OXYGEN   OXYGEN   LUNGS   OXYGEN

OXYGEN RICH BLOOD

Cardiac output increases from 5 to 25 liters/minute. Blood flow is shunted away from the intestines and other abdominal organs to the exercising muscle. (Adapted from Astrand and Rodahl, *Textbook of Work Physiology.* New York: McGraw-Hill, 1970.)

Figure 15-3.   CARDIOVASCULAR CHANGES DURING RUNNING

Testing Cardiac Function

How do we evaluate cardiac function? The nervous impulses that travel through the heart's electrical conducting system can be recorded in a doctor's office with an electrocardiogram (EKG). An EKG records the heart's electrical energy, allowing analysis of heart rate, thickness of heart muscle, abnormalities in heart rhythm and detection of areas of heart muscle with decreased blood supply (Figure 15-4).

The cardiovascular system's main purpose is to supply oxygen to body tissues. Therefore, one of the major parameters used by exercise physiologists to measure the cardiovascular system's efficiency is *oxygen consumption*. At sea level, air *inhaled* by the lungs contains 21 percent oxygen. Body tissues use some of that oxygen; thus air *exhaled* by the lungs will contain less. The oxygen difference between inhaled and exhaled air is called the body's oxygen consumption. As we exercise, muscles require more oxygen, and heart rate and stroke volume increase in order to increase the supply of oxygen-rich blood to the muscles. The body's oxygen consumption will increase until the heart reaches its maximum ability to deliver oxygen to the muscles. This *maximum oxygen consumption* reflects the maximum cardiovascular potential. The capacity of muscles to exercise while metabolizing oxygen is called *aerobic work*.

There is an obvious relationship between maximum oxygen consumption and the ability to perform aerobic work such as long distance running. Maximum oxygen consumption is expressed either in terms of liters of oxygen per minute or as milliliters of oxygen per kilogram of body weight per minute. Most normal young adults range between 45–60 milliliters per kilogram per minute or about 4 liters of oxygen per minute, while world class distance runners range between 70–80 milliliters per kilogram per minute or 6 liters of oxygen per minute.

Training the Cardiovascular System

How does running affect the cardiovascular system? The main alterations are increase in stroke volume, change in resting heart

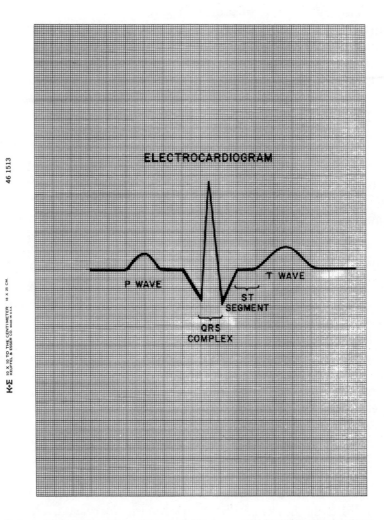

Detects electrical impulses of heart. P Wave = atrial (small) heart chambers. QRS Complex = ventricles (major) heart chambers. T Wave = repolarization of electrical impulse.

Figure 15-4. ELECTROCARDIOGRAM (EKG)

rate and alterations in blood flow to exercising muscles (Figure 15-5). Stroke volume of well-trained runners is 1½–2 times normal. This is a result of enlargement of heart muscle fibers, as well as dilation of the heart's internal pumping chamber. The heart becomes a larger, more powerful pump, and cardiac output is increased.

Maximum heart rate is not affected by training. Rather, this is a gift of nature that slowly declines with age. Resting heart rate, however, is lowered by training, partly due to increased stroke volume, but more important, because of alterations in nervous tone which controls heart rate.

One of the major results of training is increased blood flow to exercising muscles. New networks of blood vessels grow to supply muscle groups being exercised. In addition, enzymatic changes occur in trained muscle (described in Chapter 4). The end result of these two alterations is the so-called peripheral effect, which yields greater efficiency in the delivery of oxygen-rich blood to exercising muscles because the muscles can extract more oxygen from the blood. An added benefit is general decrease in nervous tone of the blood vessels resulting in a desirable decrease in blood pressure at rest.

Alterations in the cardiovascular system due to training are summarized in Figure 15-6. Increased stroke volume results in increased cardiac output. Alteration in blood vessel supply to exercising muscles and enzymatic changes both result in increased oxygen extraction by exercising muscles. These effects lead to increased maximum oxygen consumption and, as a result, increased maximum work capacity or increased aerobic capacity. However, an increase in efficiency of oxygen consumption during submaximal exercise is just as important. In other words, because of increased efficiency in the delivery and utilization of oxygen, the cardiac work load is decreased. These benefits are best reflected in the heart rate. For example, the pulse of an untrained person may be 70 at rest and 160 while running a 7-minute mile. After training, the pulse may be 50 at rest and increase to only 130 during the same 7-minute mile. Similarly, a trained individual can run faster with the same amount of cardiac work. Before training, a person running at 75 percent of his maximum heart rate might average a 7-minute mile, while max-

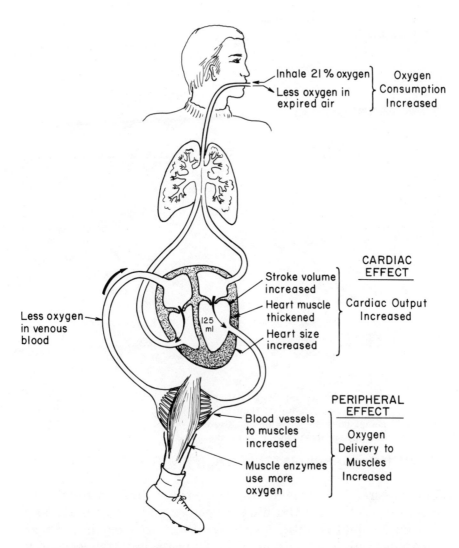

Inhale 21 % oxygen
Less oxygen in expired air
Oxygen Consumption Increased

CARDIAC EFFECT
Stroke volume increased
Heart muscle thickened
Heart size increased
Cardiac Output Increased

125 ml

Less oxygen in venous blood

PERIPHERAL EFFECT
Blood vessels to muscles increased
Muscle enzymes use more oxygen
Oxygen Delivery to Muscles Increased

Training effects on the heart include increased stroke volume, thickened heart muscle and a low resting heart rate. The result is a larger heart which is a more efficient pump (runners' heart). Peripheral effects from training include the development of new blood vessels in muscle and extraction of more oxygen from blood by muscle enzymes. Result is increased oxygen delivery to muscle cells.

Figure 15-5. TRAINING THE CARDIOVASCULAR SYSTEM

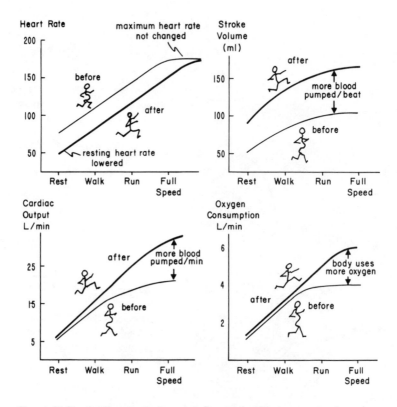

(Top, left) Resting heart rate lowered. Runner is able to run at submaximum speed with lower heart rate. (Top, right) Stroke volume increased. (Bottom, left) Heart pumps more blood per minute. (Bottom, right) Increased oxygen consumption. Body is able to use more oxygen.

Figure 15-6.   CARDIOVASCULAR ALTERATIONS WITH TRAINING

imum heart rate and maximum oxygen consumption might yield a 6-minute mile. After training, 75 percent of the maximum heart rate might yield a 6-minute mile, while the same maximum heart rate will result in a 5-minute mile. Thus, the heart rate needed to perform a fixed amount of work is lowered.

Cardiovascular Problems

CORONARY ARTERY DISEASE

The most common disease affecting the heart is coronary artery disease. This usually develops when fatty deposits build up inside the coronary arteries, causing narrowing of the internal diameter. The fatty buildup is called *atherosclerosis.* When the internal diameter of the coronary arteries is sufficiently reduced, the body is no longer able to supply oxygen-rich blood to cardiac muscles, and the heart is forced to work without adequate oxygen to meet its metabolic needs.

There are basically three degrees of coronary artery disease. In the first stage there are no clinical symptoms, but an electrocardiogram (EKG) will indicate *decreased coronary blood flow* either at rest or during exercise. During a so-called stress test which is usually performed on a treadmill, an EKG constantly monitors heart activity as a patient exercises. Work load is gradually intensified by increasing the speed and incline of the treadmill. Coronary artery disease can be suspected when abnormalities occur, such as irregular or abnormally fast heart rate, depression of the EKG baseline indicating ischemia (low blood flow), or an abnormal rise in blood pressure (see Figure 15-7). Although the stress test is not always entirely accurate, it does generally detect most cases of coronary artery disease. Since many elite runners also have abnormal stress tests, the test is probably not of much value in highly trained athletes.

More severe coronary artery disease may result in the second stage: *angina pectoris,* which is Latin for chest pain. When heart muscle is deprived of oxygen, pain can develop. The pain usually occurs under conditions of emotional or physical stress when the heart rate and work load are increased, raising cardiac oxygen needs. Narrow coronary arteries are unable to supply enough blood to heart muscle, causing a fall in the heart's oxygen level. The pain that results may be a squeezing cramplike pain or dull burning pressure in the mid-chest or back. Pain may be present in the jaw or cause numbness of either arm or fingers. Sometimes angina causes nausea and stomach discomfort, leading to a mistaken diagnosis of indigestion. These symptoms usually disappear within a few minutes after exertion stops and heart rate slows.

The most severe manifestation, the third stage, of coronary artery disease is a *heart attack or myocardial infarction.* In this instance, a coronary artery is completely blocked by fatty accumulation or blod clot. Heart muscle dependent upon blood from a blocked coronary artery will die within a few hours because of

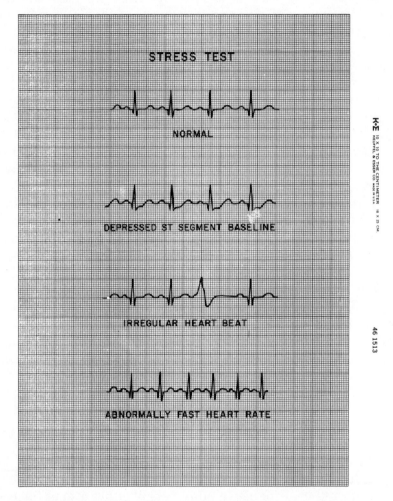

The three most common abnormal patterns (depressed ST segment, irregular heartbeat, and abnormally fast heart rate) may indicate low blood flow to heart as a result of narrow coronary arteries.

Figure 15-7. ELECTROCARDIOGRAM PERFORMED DURING EXERCISE (STRESS TEST)

lack of oxygen. The severity of a heart attack depends upon the amount of cardiac muscle that dies and whether or not the heart's normal electrical system is interrupted with a *cardiac arrest* or *ventricular fibrillation*. Cardiac arrest means that the heart completely stops beating. Ventricular fibrillation means that heart muscle contractions are completely disorganized. In both instances, no blood is pumped to the body and death occurs in minutes. Immediate medical attention can reverse a cardiac arrest or ventricular fibrillation. If a patient survives a heart attack, scar tissue will replace the area of dead heart muscle. This will usually result in some weakening of the pumping action of the heart, once again relative to the degree of involved heart muscle.

A patient does not always progress from early stages of coronary artery disease through angina pectoris to a heart attack. Some individuals will feel completely normal until their first heart attack. Conversely, other people will have angina pectoris for years without ever developing a full-blown myocardial infarction.

Cause: More people in the United States die from coronary artery disease than from any other cause. Despite this fact, medical science is still unsure of many basic mechanisms contributing to coronary artery disease. But studies of patients and various populations of people have revealed certain risk factors. The chance of heart attack increases with high blood pressure, cigarette smoking, obesity, inherited tendency to coronary artery disease, diabetes, high blood cholesterol and other fats, emotional stress, aggressive personality type and physical inactivity. Males have a higher incidence than females. Epidemiologists who study groups of people have implicated all of these elements and indicate that cigarette smoking, high blood pressure and high blood fats are probably the most important risk factors for the average American.

Of particular interest to runners is the role of exercise in the prevention of coronary artery disease. A variety of studies have indicated that physically active people have a lower death rate from coronary artery disease. Primitive people who exercise daily and eat sparingly are remarkably free of the disease. Examples include: African Masai tribesmen who tend goats on foot; Mexican Tarahumara Indians who travel 10–20 miles daily and engage in long distance football (soccer) games during which they run over 100 miles; and long-lived Soviet Georgians who also cover miles on foot each day. Population studies of western man compared active versus sedentary people, including London bus conductors versus bus drivers, American mail carriers versus mail clerks, train switchmen versus railroad clerks, manual laborers versus desk workers and college oarsmen versus nonathletic classmates. While there is still considerable debate as to the exact validity and implication of these studies, most investigators do conclude that physically active people have less coronary artery disease and lower death rates from heart attacks.

Some physicians carry these correlations to the extreme by stating that trained marathon runners do not die of atherosclerotic-induced heart attacks. They point to the protective effect of changes in body fats that occur among long distance runners, and enlargement of coronary arteries noted at autopsy of marathon runners such as the famous Boston marathoner, Clarence DeMar, whose coronary arteries were three times normal size when he died of cancer at the age of sixty-nine. While these claims are intriguing, only further study will prove whether or not marathon running causes complete or partial immunity to coronary artery disease. Runners are not immortal, and heart attacks have been well documented among those who run less than the marathon distance.

Symptoms and Diagnosis: Many individuals with coronary artery disease are totally unaware that they have a problem. When their hearts are stressed with unusual exertion such as running, symptoms may become evident. In some instances, angina pectoris will occur, while occasionally more severe complications and even sudden death may ensue. Every year a few people die suddenly during heavy physical exertion such as shoveling snow, lifting heavy objects and even jogging. Should this be of undue concern to the average runner? The answer is emphatically No! But a sensible approach is warranted. People over the age of thirty who take up jogging or running for the first time or after a long period of inactivity should be checked by their physician before starting an exercise program. After a routine physical examination, an electrocardiogram and stress test will probably be performed. While the stress test is not foolproof, it will help identify many of those people who are at risk.

Even when the examination and stress test are normal, a beginning runner should proceed gradually into a training program. It takes time for the body, and especially the heart, to adjust to the extra effort required by running. Generally, a beginner should aim to sustain his heart rate at 70–80 percent of his predicted maximum (Figure 15-8) during a workout. It's almost impossible to take your pulse while running. Check your pulse after you've run for 10 minutes at a steady pace. Stop running and place your index finger on your pulse, which is along the

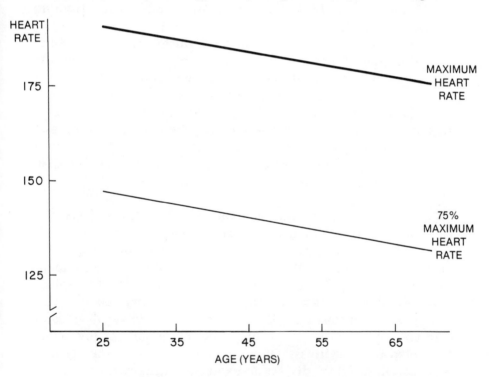

Maximum heart rate slowly declines with age and is not affected by training. Goal of running rehabilitation program is to exercise at approximately 75 percent of maximum heart rate for 30 minutes at least three times a week.

Figure 15-8.   TARGET PULSE

side of your wrist below your thumb. Count the number of beats for the first 15 seconds and multiply by 4. Each week the duration, but not the speed, of running should be increased. Running at this intensity for one-half hour three times a week is about the minimum required for beneficial cardiovascular effects.

There are two main aspects of coronary artery disease to remember. First, be aware of the symptoms of coronary artery disease and the appropriate tests and precautions that should be taken. Second, people with documented coronary artery disease must take very special care when starting a running program. Warning signs of heart disease are:

1. Pain or discomfort in the chest, back, jaw, left shoulder, either arm or upper abdomen while running. These symptoms may develop at the start of a run and gradually disappear or may be present only under levels of high stress such as hill running or speed workouts.

2. Irregular pulse or fluttering heart during or after running.

3. Episodes of racing heart while resting or exercising mildly.

Runners who suspect trouble should seek help. Even if a stress test indicates silent coronary artery disease, do not despair. There is evidence that a running program may be one of the best ways to prevent the progression of early coronary artery disease. But people who do have abnormal tests should proceed with caution and enroll themselves in a medically supervised cardiac exercise program when they begin their training.

Comments and Treatment: The treatment of coronary artery disease has changed drastically over the past twenty-five years. After a heart attack, physical exercise of any kind used to be taboo. Most people with heart disease were strictly forbidden, for life, to engage in any type of strenuous activity. But epidemiologic studies suggested that, to the contrary, people who engaged in vigorous exercise seemed to have lower degrees of coronary artery disease. This tantalizing bit of evidence prompted pioneer investigators to cautiously encourage people with coronary artery disease to exercise. Initial results were so promising that the pendulum has swung in the opposite direction, and during the past ten years there has been an enormous expansion of exercise programs for people with coronary artery disease. While there is still controversy among cardiologists as to the exact role of exercise in treatment of the disease, there is no longer any doubt that these programs are beneficial for many patients.

The basic goal of exercise therapy for people with coronary artery disease is to improve their aerobic capacity. When the body's exercise oxygen consumption in increased, there is less stress on the heart. Running is the foundation of almost all exercise therapy programs. Patients are closely supervised as exercise is gradually increased. The goal is to exercise for approximately one-half hour three times a week at a capacity of approximately 60–75 percent of the maximum aerobic ability. Remember that oxygen consumption is directly related to the heart rate. If a patient's maximum heart rate is 170, therefore, the target exercise should cause a pulse rate of 130–140 in order to reflect an oxygen consumption of approximately 75 percent of maximum (see Figure 15-8).

How do running programs benefit people with coronary artery disease? Increased aerobic power usually occurs, which means that the heart's workload during exercise decreases. This benefit is similar to the training effect outlined above. Additional advantages include: decreased blood pressure, decreased resting heart rate, decreased cholesterol and body fat, and decreased weight. A large number of patients with angina pectoris will note decrease in severity or total absence of these symptoms. While there is still some debate, most physicians think there is also some reduction in mortality rate, particularly in those patients who continue regular exercise.

How does exercise training help coronary artery disease? Most of the benefits appear to be secondary to peripheral changes rather than alterations in the coronary arteries or the heart muscle itself. There is usually not much improvement in cardiac stroke volume because of underlying disease of the heart muscle. Blood vessels in the exercising muscles decrease their tone, allowing better muscle blood flow. Alterations of muscle enzymes that utilize oxygen mean increased oxygen uptake from the blood. There is probably little or no change in the blood flow through the coronary arteries or the strength of the heart muscle. Some investigators claim that new blood vessels called *collaterals* develop in the heart muscle, but this is not a well-documented finding.

Individuals who complete the training period also note increased ability to work, increased stamina and capacity for exercise, decreased heart symptoms with normal activity, improved psychological outlook, decreased need for cardiac medication and increased sexual performance, stamina and capacity. These results certainly appear worth the effort. Some doctors, however, point to certain drawbacks of exercise therapy. There are some clearly defined risks to be considered. A high dropout rate noted in most programs indicates that a large number of patients are unable to obtain the desired benefits. Some individuals even suffer increased symptoms which are usually associated with progressive heart disease. Cardiac arrest may occur during an exercise program, although the incidence of these episodes is low (a few percent) and most patients are successfully resuscitated by attending doctors. If a patient exercises under closely supervised conditions, the risk of sudden death is minimal. Musculoskeletal problems frequently develop in sedentary individuals who enroll in exercise programs, but they are usually minor and gradually disappear.

One of the most important criticisms of exercise therapy programs is that the high expectations touted by enthusiasts are beyond the limits of many patients. Those people who benefit most from exercise programs are those with mild or moderate disease. Many people with more severe disease, particularly older people, have too much scar tissue in the heart or such severe narrowing of the coronary arteries that it is virtually impossible for them to benefit from exercise training. Unfortunately, this group of patients includes a large percentage of the American population.

How do exercise programs compare with other kinds of treatment for coronary artery disease? There are two other types of therapy generally considered for treatment of patients with coronary artery disease: drug therapy and bypass heart surgery. The nitrite or vasodilator group of drugs (nitroglycerine) act by dilating blood vessels, thereby decreasing the work that the heart has to perform in order to pump blood through the coronary arteries. The resultant increased aerobic power is of the same order of magnitude as that noted with exercise training programs. Vasodilator therapy may be combined with exercise therapy, leading to greater benefits. Another group of drugs frequently used are called beta-adrenergic blockade drugs. Inderal is the drug usually used. These medications decrease the heart rate and the resistance to blood flow in the arteries. Inderal, however, prevents the increase in cardiac output necessary to supply blood to exercising muscles. Many individuals taking this drug become faint, and even collapse when they attempt strenuous exercise, making Inderal and exercise a bad combination.

Coronary artery bypass surgery is a procedure by which a vein is connected to a coronary artery to shunt blood around a narrowed area of the artery and to increase blood flow to the heart. This surgery results in increased aerobic power approximately equal to both drug therapy and exercise rehabilitation. Running therapy is frequently used to supplement the benefits of bypass surgery.

RUNNER'S HEART

During training, a long distance runner's heart becomes stronger and more efficient than that of his sedentary peers. These alterations have been well studied, and there are apparently no adverse effects from the development of a runner's heart, even though these alterations superficially resemble abnormalities of a sick heart. A runner's heart is larger than normal, and there are changes in pulse rate and rhythm. A physician may hear heart murmur and note "abnormalities" of the electrocardiogram and stress test. All of these changes are also seen in diseased flabby hearts. The resemblance, however, is superficial since a runner's heart is actually a strong, healthy, efficient pump, while a diseased heart is weakened with overstressed muscle fibers and a failing pump.

The stroke volume of the larger-than-normal runner's heart will gradually increase so that more blood can be pumped with each heartbeat. Individual muscle fibers also enlarge with training. This results in cardiac enlargement which may be observed during routine physical examination, chest X ray, or electrocardiogram. (Electrocardiogram abnormalities are listed for physicians' reference in the Appendix.) There is a common misconception that when an athlete retires from competition, his large muscular heart will deteriorate into a large fatty or flabby organ. This is untrue. Studies of athletes placed on strict bed rest show that heart muscle shrinks and the overall heart size usually returns to normal within a few weeks. This change does not occur with diseased hearts.

Another common abnormality of distance runners is a heart murmur, or what are called extra cardiac sounds or gallops. These heart sounds are seen in over 50 percent of well-trained distance runners and are entirely normal. They probably reflect the strong pumping action of a runner's muscular heart.

Slow heart rate is almost universally noted among trained distance runners. Many of these athletes also have abnormalities of their hearts' nervous conducting system. These "partial heart blocks" are noted on the electrocardiogram and seem to be of no pathologic significance.

Elite long distance runners frequently have abnormal stress tests. The changes that occur are identical to abnormalities seen with coronary artery disease. When these findings are noted among patients with coronary artery disease, they are thought to indicate ischemia (low blood flow) to coronary muscle. But it is difficult to imagine that these changes represent disease of any type when they are found among some of the world's best marathon runners. When evaluating a trained distance runner, therefore, stress test interpretation is extremely difficult. Fortunately, there are even more sophisticated ways of testing for coronary artery disease when a physician thinks such procedures are necessary.

Occasionally, an unsuspecting physician will erroneously make a diagnosis of cardiac disease in a healthy runner. Runners have experienced difficulties during annual team physicals, and they have been denied life insurance out of ignorance of basic cardiac physiology. Over the years, many young runners have been barred from competition because strong, healthy, athletic hearts were mistakenly thought to be diseased. One such example is Clarence DeMar, who stopped running for several years when his doctors found "abnormalities." When a runner is told that he has heart disease, he should mention the possibility of runner's heart to his physician in order to make sure that an incorrect diagnosis is not made.

HEART MURMURS

Cause: Blood flowing past a structural abnormality of the heart causes a turbulent sound called a heart murmur. These sounds may be caused by abnormal heart valves, such as leaky, roughened or stiff cardiac valves resulting from a congenital heart disease or from rheumatic fever. However, a heart murmur can be completely innocuous, the result of the strong pumping action of a muscular heart.

Symptoms and Diagnosis: Usually there are no symptoms associated with a heart murmur. When a heart murmur represents severe disease of the heart valves, symptoms of heart failure may be present, including shortness of breath at rest or with mild exertion, rapid pulse rate and swelling of the ankles, feet and legs.

By the nature of the murmur, a physician or cardiologist can frequently determine whether a heart murmur is innocuous (functional murmur) or representative of cardiac valve disease. When matters are not so clear-cut, more extensive testing is warranted. Studies might include an electrocardiogram and an ultrasound evaluation of heart valves, in which sound waves are bounced off cardiac valves, producing a picture similar to a radar screen. This study defines many abnormalities of cardiac structure and function. If a physician is still unsatisfied, he may recommend a cardiac catheterization. During this procedure, a small plastic catheter is passed through the blood vessels into the heart's chambers. When dye is injected through the catheter, the heart valves are visualized in action and recorded on motion picture X rays. Pressures in the heart's chambers are also measured during cardiac catheterization.

Comments and Treatment: If a heart murmur is functional, it is of no importance and doctors recommend completely normal activity, including running and competition. But when structural abnormalities of the heart exist, therapy might be recommended. In extreme cases, a heart operation may be required to repair or replace damaged cardiac valves. In other cases, a cardiologist may elect medical care and long-term observation.

It is impossible to make a generalization regarding running with a diseased heart valve. While many people with mild cardiac valvular disease have competed successfully as athletes and runners, an afflicted runner should discuss his problem with a cardiologist. Each case must be reviewed individually. Because some doctors are more conservative than others, a runner who is not satisfied should not hesitate to obtain a second opinion.

IRREGULAR HEARTBEAT

Cause: Normal rhythmic heartbeat may be interrupted by sudden discharge of electrical energy from an irritable area of heart muscle. Anyone can develop irregular heartbeats at one time or another, resulting from excitement, lack of sleep or stimulants such as caffeine and nicotine. Other cases are caused by heart disease such as coronary artery disease or abnormalities of the heart's electrical conducting system.

While some studies indicate that irregular heartbeats are more common among runners, other investigations show no difference between runners and other healthy individuals. However, one type of irregular heartbeat that is probably more common in runners is called "racing heart syndrome" or supraventricular tachycardia. Heart rate will suddenly speed to almost 200 beats a minute during these attacks. Many of these cases are due to short circuit of the heart's nervous conducting system called Wolff-Parkinson-White syndrome, an abnormality that is apparently common among long distance runners.

Symptoms and Diagnosis: While many individuals with occasional irregular heartbeats have no symptoms, others will note a fluttering or flip-flop sensation in the chest. Racing heart syndrome may cause a transient fluttering or a sustained speeding of the heart, resulting in weakness and dizziness. These attacks may occur at rest or while running and may be extremely uncomfortable. They may last for only a few moments or for several hours.

If you suspect irregular heartbeat, check your own pulse. Irregular heartbeat or racing of the pulse while resting suggests this diagnosis. In that event, consult your doctor for a possible electrocardiogram, which usually indicates the cause of irregular heartbeat. In some instances, however, an EKG taken while running is necessary for diagnosis. A standard stress test may be adequate, but sometimes a monitor is attached to a runner's chest to record heartbeats on an electromagnetic tape, which can then be analyzed. An even more sophisticated method is called telemetry, a process by which a chest monitor sends continuous radio wave signals, producing an EKG on a central monitor as a runner circles a track.

Comments and Treatment: If there is frequent irregularity or racing heart, see a doctor for a possible electrocardiogram (EKG). Everyone develops an occasional irregular heartbeat, and these are probably of no consequence. Some cases, however, are more serious. The racing heart syndrome can be dangerous, and medical therapy is available to prevent attacks.

RHEUMATIC FEVER

Cause: Rheumatic fever is an inflammatory disease that occurs following streptococcal sore throat. The body's normal defenses against infection are turned against itself causing inflammation of skin, joints, nervous system and the heart. Inflammation of heart muscle (myocarditis) is a serious problem that can cause heart failure. Heart valves are also frequently inflamed, and over a period of years, these damaged valves become scarred and roughened, frequently resulting in chronic cardiac valvular disease and heart murmurs.

Children and adolescents are particularly prone to rheumatic fever. In fact, approximately 5 percent of people under age twenty-five who have a strep throat will develop rheumatic fever. Epidemics of streptococcal sore throat in a classroom or institutional setting are common in school-age children.

Symptoms and Diagnosis: A few weeks after a strep throat, symptoms will develop, including a rash, joint pains, bumps or nodules under the skin, nervous twitches called chorea, and inflammation of the heart and heart valves. Myocarditis may cause cardiac weakness and failure. However, the vast majority of cases are not detected, and the individual is unaware that he is sustaining damage to his heart. Only years later do symptoms of malfunctioning cardiac valves become apparent.

A physician can make a diagnosis of rheumatic fever on the basis of a physical evaluation, an electrocardiogram, and blood tests indicating a recent streptococcal infection.

Comments and Treatment: A large percentage of cases of rheumatic fever can be avoided if streptococcal sore throat is treated promptly with adequate doses of antibiotics such as penicillin. For this reason, a young person who develops sore throat should seek medical attention for a throat culture and possible diagnosis of strep throat. If strep is found, penicillin should be taken for 10 days.

If an unfortunate runner does develop rheumatic fever, rest is absolutely mandatory. Vigorous exercise during acute myocarditis may lead to severe damage and even heart failure.

Adult runners who have heart murmurs due to rheumatic fever of childhood should consult a cardiologist. Complete evaluation is mandatory before engaging in strenuous competition.

ATHEROSCLEROSIS—CHOLESTEROL AND BLOOD FATS

Cause: High levels of cholesterol and other fats in the blood increase the risk of coronary artery disease. These substances infiltrate blood vessel walls, causing local inflammation and thickening. Calcium is deposited on top of the fat and rock-hard plaques slowly build up on the inside of the blood vessel walls. This disease is called atherosclerosis. As a result of blood vessel narrowing, there is decreased blood flow to organs normally supplied by these arteries. Symptoms of low tissue oxygen may then occur. Examples include angina pectoris (cardiac pain due to atherosclerosis of coronary arteries) and claudication (leg pain during exercise due to atherosclerosis of leg arteries).

Cholesterol and other fats enter the blood by high dietary intake of animal fats and cholesterol and the body's normal production of cholesterol independent of dietary intake. The average American diet is particularly rich in saturated fats and cholesterol, which probably accounts for the development of atherosclerosis among many young individuals. Autopsies performed on American servicemen killed during the Korean war showed an alarmingly high rate of far advanced atherosclerosis among these eighteen to twenty-five year-old healthy young soldiers. Some people have an inherited tendency to produce excess quantities of cholesterol and other blood fats. There is usually a family history of early deaths from heart disease, stroke and other complications of atherosclerosis.

Dangerous blood fats can usually be lowered by diet, substituting foods rich in polyunsaturated fats for those containing cholesterol and saturated animal fats. Well-trained runners have a low level of cholesterol and other dangerous fats in their blood. These same runners also have an increased high-density lipoprotein fats profile. These fats, which are sometimes termed "friendly fats," do not cause atherosclerosis. On the contrary, high levels seem to offer protection against the development of atherosclerosis. Alteration of the ratio between dangerous fats and friendly fats may be one of the most beneficial aspects of long distance running and a major reason that runners rarely develop coronary artery disease.

Both diet and exercise are responsible for this healthy blood fat picture. Many runners refrain from diets high in animal fats, preferring polyunsaturated foods made with peanut oil and vegetable oil. In addition, while running the body metabolizes considerable quantities of cholesterol and dangerous fats.

Since atherosclerosis begins early in life, proper diet and exercise should start during childhood. An interesting question remains, however. Can anything be done for the adult who already suffers from atherosclerosis? Can calcium-impregnated atherosclerotic plaques regress and disappear if you change your life-style with a proper diet and long distance running? No one knows the answer. But some investigators do think that at least partial reversal of atherosclerotic plaques is possible.

Symptoms and Diagnosis: There are no specific symptoms of high cholesterol and dangerous blood fats unless these substances reach very high levels. By the time symptoms of atherosclerosis develop, the disease is usually far advanced. Those with family histories of heart disease, stroke, claudication or other atherosclerotic complications should be aware of increased risk.

Blood fat levels can be accurately measured by tests called serum cholesterol, triglycerides and lipoprotein electrophoresis. Any person with coronary artery disease or a strong family history of atherosclerosis should have these tests done. Not only do dietary changes help improve the overall picture, but in severe cases specific medications are available to lower dangerous fats.

Comments and Treatment: Most runners should be confident of a healthy blood fat picture to help prevent the ravages of atherosclerosis. Those runners who have borderline elevation of cholesterol or who wish to lower blood levels below the normal range should try a diet high in polyunsaturated fats. One food that appears of particular benefit is yogurt. African Masai tribesmen who consume very large quantities of cholesterol also have very low blood cholesterol levels. This is partly a result of vigorous physical exercise but is also probably due to their large dietary intake of yogurt. Soviet Georgians who are renowned for longevity also consume large amounts of yogurt. Recent American studies indicate that diets rich in yogurt will lower blood cholesterol within a few weeks. This substance, therefore, appears to be one of the truly beneficial "natural foods."

HIGH BLOOD PRESSURE

Cause: Hypertension remains a medical mystery even though 15 percent of adult Americans suffer from it. In a small percentage of patients, diseases such as tumors of the adrenal or pituitary glands and structural abnormalities of the aorta or blood vessels of the kidneys are found. The rest of the cases are called essential hypertension, which means that we do not know the cause. There are certain risk factors that predispose to high blood pressure such as family history, obesity, emotional stress and high salt diet. Males and blacks have a higher incidence. Hypertension begins early in life, being very common among children.

Physiologically, hypertension means elevation of the pressure in the arteries of the body. As a result, the heart must work harder to pump against this increased pressure. This eventually can lead to such complications as enlargement and ultimate failure of the heart. In addition, hypertension predisposes to atherosclerosis of the blood vessels. When the pressure is very high, blood vessel walls can weaken and rupture. Rupture of a blood vessel in the brain can result in a stroke, one of the most feared complications of hypertension.

Symptoms and Diagnosis: Since most people with hypertension are unaware that they suffer from this disease until serious damage has occurred, periodic check of blood pressure is the best insurance against complications of hypertension. This is probably the single most important routine medical procedure. Hypertension may develop at an early age, so screening should start during childhood and continue throughout life.

Comments and Treatment: Hypertension is treated with a variety of medications that lower blood vessel pressure. Endurance training such as running usually lowers blood pressure, an additional benefit to a runner's health. It is certainly advisable, therefore, for people with mild hypertension to consider a running program. However, since blood pressure rises temporarily during running, individuals with severe degrees of hypertension should check with their doctors and receive medication before starting a running program. Once blood pressure is controlled, you can safely run. One note of caution: Some antihypertensive medications can cause harmful side effects during running. Inderal, one of the newer and most effective antihypertensive drugs, is particularly troublesome because it decreases cardiac output. People who exercise strenuously while taking Inderal may become dizzy and faint. A runner should therefore take an alternative medication for control of his blood pressure and should discuss this problem thoroughly with his physician.

POSTURAL HYPOTENSION (LOW BLOOD PRESSURE)

Cause: Runners frequently develop postural hypotension, noting dizziness and partial blackouts when they stand up suddenly after sitting or lying down for a period of time. Postural hypotension is caused by temporary low blood pressure with changes in position. As a result of training, runners frequently have low blood pressure and increased activity of the vagus nerve, which predisposes them to postural hypotension. Other runners develop this symptom because they are partially dehydrated from excessive sweat loss during runs in hot weather. Although postural hypotension can be annoying and temporarily disabling, it is of no real pathologic importance.

Symptoms and Diagnosis: Dizziness, weakness and transient black spots in front of the eyes are symptoms of postural hypotension. Attacks usually occur when you get out of bed in the morning or when you suddenly stand after sitting for prolonged periods of time. These uncomfortable sensations disappear within a few moments.

A runner should confirm that the symptoms represent postural hypotension. A doctor will note changes in blood pressure as the runner moves from a lying to a standing position. Normally, blood pressure increases slightly when you stand. Significant fall in blood pressure with erect posture suggests postural hypotension.

Comments and Treatment: There is no specific treatment for postural hypotension. If you are prone to this symptom, take the precaution of rising slowly after a period of rest. If dizziness is severe, alleviate this symptom by placing your head between your legs to increase blood flow to the brain.

It should be stressed that symptoms of postural hypotension are transient, lasting only a few seconds. Runners who suffer from prolonged dizzy spells should seek medical attention for detection of more serious problems.

CHEST PAIN

Cause and Symptoms: One of the most frequent symptoms that brings a patient to a doctor is chest pain. It has many causes, some minor and others more serious. Since most runners will note some degree of pain and discomfort in the chest at one time or another, it is important to be aware of the more common causes and their symptoms.

1. *Heart disease.* Coronary artery disease can produce pain in the chest called angina pectoris (discussed earlier in chapter). Remember that pain of coronary artery disease usually occurs during exertion and disappears within 2–3 minutes after exertion ceases. If the pain lasts for more than a few minutes after exertion is discontinued, angina pectoris is unlikely. Coronary artery disease much less commonly produces pain at rest or during sleep.

2. *Pericarditis.* Inflammation of the heart's lining (the pericardium) is called pericarditis. Viral infection is the most common cause of this disease. Pain of pericarditis, which is caused by stretching of the sac surrounding the heart, is generally felt in the mid-chest or back. It is usually sharp and worsened by deep breathing, coughing or other movements of the lungs and diaphragm. People with more advanced cases of pericarditis may experience shortness of breath. Symptoms of viral illness such as fever, nasal congestion and cough are frequently present.

3. *Pleurisy.* Inflammation of the lining of the lungs (pleura) is called pleuritis of pleurisy. Viral infection is the most common cause. Sharp pain is usually felt in the chest wall or the shoulders and is aggravated by deep breathing. Fever, cough and other influenza-type symptoms are frequently present.

4. *Costochondritis.* Inflammation of the joints connecting the ribs to the breast bone is called costochondritis. This may result from a minor injury to the chest wall or may be associated with heavy strenuous exercise. Pain is usually localized to an area along the margin of the breast bone where minor swelling and redness are sometimes noted. There are usually no other symptoms of disease.

5. *Degenerative arthritis.* Irregularities of body joints frequently develop with age. This disease, which is called degenerative or osteoarthritis, is discussed in Chapter 20. Arthritis of the neck or shoulder frequently causes pain radiating down to the chest or arms. This type of pain is usually sharp and can be constant or shooting in character. Symptoms are frequently aggravated by movement of the shoulders or neck.

6. *Spontaneous pneumothorax.* Sudden rupture of a small air

sac in the lung is called spontaneous pneumothorax. Young athletes, including runners, frequently develop this condition. Symptoms begin suddenly, often developing during heavy exertion. Severe chest and shoulder pain aggravated by breathing and sometimes accompanied by shortness of breath is noted.

7. *Musculoskeletal pain.* A strain or pull of a muscle of the chest wall may occur during heavy physical exertion. This type of pain, which is usually sharp and persistent, is aggravated by twisting the body and breathing deeply. Local tenderness of the involved muscle is frequent.

8. *Gastrointestinal disease.* Pain in the chest can result from disease of the esophagus, stomach, small intestine, or gallbladder. These diseases are described in Chapter 16. Gastrointestinal pain is usually dull or burning and felt in the area of the breast bone or lower chest. Nausea, vomiting, and belching are frequent.

Diagnosis: There are a wide variety of conditions that cause chest pain and an even wider number of tests used for diagnosis. A physician can usually narrow the possibilities by careful history and physical examination. Further tests, such as chest X ray, electrocardiogram, stress test, or X rays of the gastrointestinal tract, may then be requested.

Comments and Treatment: A runner must frequently decide whether discomfort in his chest is a symptom of disease rather than normal result of vigorous exertion required of speed work and road racing. The following questions should serve as a guideline:

1. Is the chest pain a new symptom not previously present under similar racing or workout conditions?

2. Is the pain so severe that it interferes with normal running and workout routines?

3. Are there associated symptoms such as weight loss, nausea, fever, cough or other conditions that may indicate a disease process?

4. Is the chest pain chronic, lasting more than a few days?

If the answer to any of these questions is Yes, seek medical attention for accurate diagnosis and proper treatment. Unfortunately, many runners are too stoical, thinking that pain is necessary or even desirable to improve racing performance. This is nonsense. It may be necessary to incur some discomfort during speed work in order to improve anaerobic running capacity. But running with pain from injury or disease usually aggravates the abnormal condition, adversely affects running form, increases risk of other injuries and threatens conditioning due to breakdown rather than buildup of muscle protein.

VARICOSE VEINS

Cause: The journey between the feet and the heart, which is the farthest distance that blood must travel in the body, is made through two networks of blood vessels: the deep and the superficial leg veins. In addition, this blood must overcome the force of gravity. For these reasons, pressure within leg veins is relatively high. Small valves line these veins to facilitate the movement of blood by preventing back flow. Occasionally, the leg vein walls weaken and the valves leak. This results in bulging, tortuous veins frequently evident on the thighs or legs, especially when standing.

People who spend the day standing or who are overweight frequently develop varicose veins. Others have an inherited tendency to develop varicose veins. Most experts think that vigorous exercise of leg muscles minimizes the development of varicose veins because the massaging effect of exercise facilitates flow of blood in the veins.

Symptoms and Diagnosis: Varicose veins usually represent a cosmetic problem. But some individuals develop inflammation of these veins, called phlebitis, which may be associated with pain and complications such as the development of blood clots.

The appearance of varicose veins varies considerably. Severe cases cause an unsightly venous pattern covering much of the leg. Milder cases may be localized to one or two small areas. These local bulges become more evident when filled with blood from standing.

Comments and Treatment: Running usually helps minimize symptoms associated with varicose veins. Support stockings, which may be custom fitted at a surgical supply house, often help those individuals who spend most of the day standing.

Phlebitis or pain from varicose veins should be treated by a vascular surgeon who will determine the severity of the disease present and might recommend either support stockings or removal of diseased veins. This surgical procedure is called venous stripping.

sweat losses that occur during hard running, even under hot conditions. However, the longer that water is retained in the stomach before it empties into the small intestine, the longer it will take to reach the body's circulation. Substances such as fats, proteins, carbohydrates and salt can drastically reduce gastric emptying of water into the small intestine, thus delaying the absorption of this much needed nutrient. Solutions containing salt and sugar, such as "aid drinks," frequently delay gastric emptying, instead of speeding up absorption, and may even cause accumulation of fluids in the stomach, resulting in cramps and nausea.

Once water gets into the small intestine, the speed with which it will diffuse across the intestinal wall is relative to the tonicity (percent of salt and sugar) of the bowel versus that of the blood. If a runner consumes an aid drink or so-called isotonic solution that contains salt or sugar, there will be an increased percentage of these substances in the bowel, and the absorption of water will be further delayed. In the extreme case, these solutions may be even more concentrated than normal body fluids, actually causing water to come out of the body into the bowel. Instead of gaining water, the body has lost some more of this precious fluid.

Water is the *most important* element that requires replacement during long distance running. Nothing must jeopardize or delay its replacement. The addition of any other substance to ingested water delays the time required for the water to get into the body. If a runner thinks that he needs sugar or salt replacement during a long run (this point is debatable), very dilute sugar and salt solutions are best (see Chapter 18).

Gastrointestinal Changes During Exercise

During exercise, blood flow is diverted away from the intestine to exercising muscle, thereby delaying digestive processes. Normal muscular contractions of the stomach and gastric emptying are inhibited, leading to retention of stomach contents. In addition, large bowel motility often increases during running, causing rapid transit of bowel contents and decreased absorption of water by the colon. These factors contribute to the cramps and diarrhea that many runners experience during or after long distance runs.

Many runners spend a great deal of time worrying about their bowels. Some of the "gastrointestinal gurus" advise fasting or ingesting only liquids the day before a race "to rest the bowel." Others recommend laxatives or enemas preceeding a race in order to remove "unneeded" fecal bulk. Much of this advice is physiologically unsound. Fasting may lead to depletion of muscle carbohydrate which is important for muscle energy during distance races. Liquid diets, laxatives, and enemas may cause diarrhea, resulting in loss of precious water and salt from the body prior to a race. Not only can this drastically impede performance, but it can also cause dehydration and heatstroke.

The most sound advice regarding racing and the bowels is this: Stick to a normal diet until the night prior to competition. Breakfast is a matter of individual preference. Heavy meals, however, should not be taken for at least 2½–3 hours prior to a race. Many foods remain in the stomach for hours, and therefore, many veterans fast the day of the race. Plain water or water containing very low concentrations of salt or sugar drunk before racing will help keep up with sweat losses during competition. During a race, plain cold water is superior to any other fluid replacement.

The gastrointestinal system undergoes no specific adaptations during training.

Gastrointestinal Problems

NAUSEA AND VOMITING

Cause: Nausea and vomiting can result from physical diseases as well as from psychic stress and emotional factors. These symptoms are mediated by a "vomiting center" in the brain, which is triggered by nervous impulses arising from different parts of the body.

Many runners note nausea and vomiting during races, particularly during the latter parts of marathons. Other unfortunate individuals note these symptoms during routine daily runs. The factors probably responsible include: decreased blood flow to the intestine and retention of food in the stomach during exercise; buildup of acid and metabolic products in the blood; and overactivity of the vagus and sympathetic nervous systems which stimulate the vomiting center.

Many runners also experience a syndrome called post-exertion nausea. Transient nausea and even retching occur immediately after a hard race. This is a normal reaction to strenuous exertion and of no serious consequence. The symptoms usually pass within a few minutes.

Symptoms and Diagnosis: Nausea and vomiting due to running may begin insidiously or may suddenly overwhelm a runner during or after a race. Chills, dizziness and cold sweat are common. Symptoms before a race are usually from "pre-race nerves." When you experience nausea or vomiting not associated with running, or if there are other symptoms such as abdominal pain, weight loss or fatigue, there may be an underlying disease such as gallbladder disease or peptic ulcers. A physician will probably order X rays of the gallbladder and gastrointestinal tract.

Comments and Treatment: Try various experiments to control your symptoms. Fasting the day of a race will minimize stomach contents. Sometimes antacids which neutralize stomach acidity are helpful. Many runners obtain relief from antihistamines (Dramamine) or parasympathetic blocking agents (Pro-Banthene) which work by blocking the vomiting center. They may be tried alone or in combination, but always experiment first during practice runs since medications affect different individuals in different ways, and it is always wise to know how your body will respond *before* a big race.

DIARRHEA, CRAMPS AND BLOATING

Cause and Symptoms: There are many diseases that cause diarrhea, and most people suffer from this problem at one time or another. It is particularly frequent among runners because vigorous exercise speeds up the bowel. This physiological reaction to exercise aggravates other underlying conditions that cause diarrhea. Be aware of the most common types of diarrhea: nervous diarrhea, irritable bowel syndrome, lactose intolerance, gluten intolerance, travelers' diarrhea, viral gastroenteritis and food allergy. Food poisoning, another cause of runners' diarrhea, is discussed in Chapter 13.

Diarrhea usually results from decreased water absorption by the bowel. Three basic mechanisms cause excess water in the stool:

1. Hypermotility or overactive bowel muscle may lead to rapid transit of intestinal contents through the bowel, leaving inadequate time for absorption. Nervous diarrhea, irritable bowel syndrome and runners' diarrhea are all Type 1.

Nervous diarrhea results from spasm of bowel muscle. Anxiety produces nervous stimulation of the bowel's smooth muscle. Runners often experience nausea and lower abdominal cramps immediately prior to a race. These discomforting symptoms usually disappear as soon as the starting gun fires when nervous energy is directed to the task of running.

The irritable bowel syndrome is extremely common among young adults, although its pathogenesis is unclear. Some authorities think emotions and allergy both play a role. The bowel's normal motility becomes irregular, and people with irritable bowel syndrome complain of bloating, lower abdominal cramps, constipation or diarrhea, and passage of mucus in the stool. These attacks occur periodically and may be aggravated by exercise, nervous tension and various foods.

Runners' diarrhea usually results from severe exercise-induced bowel hypermotility. Some runners experience these symptoms only on rare occasions, while others suffer daily attacks. These highly susceptible people may actually have another unrecognized problem such as lactose intolerance or irritable bowel syndrome.

2. Ingested food may be unabsorbable and therefore pass through the intestine carrying water with it. Lactose intolerance and gluten intolerance are Type 2.

Lactose is a sugar present in milk and dairy products. Some individuals lack an enzyme necessary to digest lactose prior to intestinal absorption. As a result, lactose remains in the bowel causing diarrhea. In extreme cases, nausea, watery stools, abdominal distention, cramps and bloating occur within an hour after drinking milk or eating dairy products. This is a relatively common problem, particularly among Jews, Orientals and Blacks. The attacks usually cease when dairy products are avoided.

Gluten is a protein present in wheat, rye, oats and barley. When susceptible people ingest gluten, degeneration of the small intestine's lining occurs, resulting in loss of normal salt and water absorption. Diarrhea, vitamin deficiency and even malnutrition may result. Because people with this disease are unable to absorb fat properly, their stools are often bulky, gray in color and float in water. The disease, which is also called idiopathic sprue or celiac disease, is inherited, occurring in approximately 1 in 2500 white Americans. It is very rare in other races.

3. Certain diseases block intestinal enzymes. As a result, water is secreted into the small bowel rather than absorbed into the body. Infections such as dysentery, viral gastroenteritis and travelers' diarrhea are Type 3.

Runners who are fortunate enough to visit foreign countries may develop travelers' diarrhea or "Montezuma's revenge." This problem frequently afflicts Olympic and national teams and can devastate a trained athlete, ruining his chances for competition. Severe cramps and diarrhea develop within a few days after arrival in a foreign country and may last for several weeks thereafter. The unfortunate victims note weakness and fatigue associated with dehydration. Most cases of travelers' diarrhea are caused by infection of the intestines by pathogenic bacteria ingested in water or food. These bacteria cause the small bowel to lose water, often resulting in severe dehydration. Persistent travelers' diarrhea may be due to intestinal parasites called amoebae or Giardia.

Viral gastroenteritis, or stomach flu, is an infection of the intestine with a virus. This illness is usually spread by close personal contact and sometimes occurs in summer epidemics. Vomiting and diarrhea occur, often in association with fever and muscle aches. Recovery usually occurs within a few days.

Food allergy is the most common cause of chronic diarrhea of infants and young children. Medical authorities still debate the importance of food allergy among adults. Almost any food can cause an allergic reaction resulting in diarrhea. But milk products, wheat, spicy foods, citrus fruits and chocolate are the most common offenders. Sometimes a clear-cut relationship between gastrointestinal symptoms and ingestion of specific foods will help pinpoint the problem. Complicated cases require medical attention and sophisticated tests such as stool analysis for parasites and fat, X rays of the intestines, lactose tolerance tests and even intestinal biopsy. Food allergy probably causes hypermotility of the bowel (Type 1 reaction) as well as fluid loss from swollen intestinal walls (Type 3 reaction).

Food allergy characteristically causes bloating, nausea, lower abdominal cramps and diarrhea within 4 hours after ingestion of the offending food. Asthma, itchy throat, hives and occasional swelling of the airways may also occur. Individuals with this disease usually have no bowel problems when they avoid allergenic food.

Comments and Treatment: Runners who suffer from hypermotility of the bowel should experiment with various approaches to the problem. Avoidance of food for several hours prior to a run often minimizes symptoms, particularly when bloating is a major component. Antispasmodics (Pro-Banthene) relax smooth muscle and decrease bowel contractions. This same medication may help severe cases of nervous diarrhea and irritable bowel. However, a runner should try this drug during light practice since unpleasant side effects such as dryness of the mouth and blurred vision may result. Bulk laxatives such as bran frequently help these three conditions. These runners should also avoid foods such as coffee, alcohol, and spices that increase bowel motility.

Lactose intolerance and gluten intolerance are treated by avoidance of lactose and gluten respectively. While this requires careful attention to the diet, the results are worth the effort.

Travelers' diarrhea is one of the major problems facing international athletes. Many competitions have been lost because of this disease. Any change from an individual's normal diet can upset the bowels and cause diarrhea. Travelers' diarrhea can be prevented or minimized by administration of antibiotics (tetracycline) starting a day before departure. Athletes should consult their team physician before international trips, particularly to South American and underdeveloped areas. They should also avoid unbottled water, raw fruits and vegetables and all uncooked food. The German national team recognizes the danger of travelers' diarrhea, and when their athletes compete in a foreign country, they are not allowed to eat any local food. All meals are prepared from food flown directly from Germany.

Athletes who note chronic diarrhea after returning home from foreign countries should have their stools analyzed for parasites.

STITCHES

Cause: Runners frequently develop abdominal pains during workouts and races. These "stitches" can be temporarily disabling. Many diseases of the chest (see Chapter 14) and abdomen (see later in chapter) can produce pain during running. The term stitch, however, is reserved for transient pain in the upper abdomen or side which develops during running and which is not due to specific internal disease. It has several causes but spasm of diaphragmatic or abdominal muscles and gas trapped in the bowel are the most common ones. There are probably other less well-recognized factors, and it has been theorized that breathing patterns and running form play a role. Untrained individuals are more prone to stitches. But athletic conditioning is no guarantee against these symptoms, and many highly trained runners suffer from stitches.

Symptoms and Diagnosis: Stitches can occur at any time during a run, but they are usually more common during the first 10–15 minutes. Veteran runners most frequently develop stitches during maximum efforts such as interval training, hill work and difficult races. Stabbing or pulling pain is felt below the rib cage, in the side and occasionally in the shoulder. These symptoms usually clear within a few moments after running is stopped. If they don't, or if pain occurs at rest, other diseases should be suspected.

Comments and Treatment: If you develop stitches during a workout, rest until the pain disappears. Walking, deep breathing, abdominal stretching exercises and sit-ups have all been reported to help.

During a race, decide for yourself whether or not to continue competing by "running through the pain." Many runners are able to overcome stitches by momentarily slowing their pace or by consciously altering their breathing pattern. Try deep breaths with violent forced expiration. In other instances, the best approach is to stop running for a few moments until the pain subsides.

Carbonated beverages frequently cause stitches and should be avoided during races.

HERNIA

Cause: The abdominal muscles normally protect the intestines. Sometimes a local weak spot develops in the abdominal wall, allowing a portion of bowel to protrude between the muscles. This condition is called hernia and occurs most frequently in the inguinal (groin region). Other sites include the femoral (upper inner thighs) and the umbilical (around the belly button) regions.

Hernias are quite common among young people who are born with weak spots of the abdominal wall. Some hernias, however, develop from excessive strain or injury to the abdominal muscles. They are most common in men.

Symptoms and Diagnosis: Many people are unaware that they have a hernia. They may note a small lump or mild discomfort or dragging in the groin. Some will experience a sudden bulge in the groin while straining or exercising. This bulge often appears and disappears. Pain may be present at first, but it usually subsides.

If you note these symptoms, consult your physician who can usually make the diagnosis by examination.

Comments and Treatment: Virtually millions of people in this country have or will develop a hernia at some time during their lives. Thousands die each year from hernia complications, the most feared of which is strangulation, occurring when abdominal muscles squeeze off the herniated bowel's blood supply, killing this portion of the intestine. Severe infection usually develops. A strangulated hernia is an emergency that requires surgical repair.

Before the development of modern surgical techniques, many hernias were treated with trusses, firm support devices that push the hernia back into the abdominal cavity. This device does not cure a hernia and does not prevent strangulation.

The modern treatment of hernia is surgical repair of a weak abdominal wall before complications develop. This operation is relatively simple and approximately 95 percent successful. Virtually all medical authorities agree that healthy people with hernias should be treated surgically. Runners who develop hernias frequently note discomfort while running and usually seek medical advice early.

HEMORRHOIDS

Cause: Enlargement of veins in the rectal region is a common condition known as piles or hemorrhoids. Predisposing factors include constipation, inactivity, hereditary weakness of the veins, straining with defecation, heavy lifting, long periods of standing, chronic diarrhea and pregnancy.

Symptoms and Diagnosis: Symptoms vary from mild discomfort to severe pain. Bleeding, local swelling around the rectum, pain and itching are common. While hemorrhoids are rarely life threatening, they lead to two complications: anemia or low red blood cell count resulting from chronic or severe bleeding hemorrhoids, and blood clotting inside swollen hemorrhoids, a condition called acute thrombosis. Swelling and extreme pain are noted around the rectum. Hard, tender "piles" are present. The pain subsides over several days, but local swelling may continue for weeks. Hemorrhoids are easily diagnosed by a physician.

Comments and Treatment: Running does not cause hemorrhoids. On the contrary, some authorities claim that running improves hemorrhoid symptoms. Because hemorrhoids are an extremely common condition, however, many runners do suffer from them, and their symptoms can certainly interfere with your enjoyment and race performance.

If you develop a mild case, treat it with witch hazel compresses applied to the hemorrhoids, and frequent warm baths. Low residue diets, mild laxatives and stool softeners help control hemorrhoid symptoms. Chronic recurrent cases as well as thrombosed hemorrhoids should be treated by a surgeon. Simple surgical repair is almost always curative.

HIATUS HERNIA

A portion of the stomach that intrudes into the chest cavity through a weak spot in the muscular diaphragm between the abdominal and chest cavities is called a hiatus hernia. Irritation of the lower esophagus can occur, resulting in heartburn and pain in the lower chest. Most cases can be treated with antacids and bland diets. Hiatus hernias are not uncommon; they rarely strangulate and most cases do not require surgery. Runners suffering from heartburn or frequent belching while running may have a hiatus hernia and should try a small glass of milk or some liquid antacid before running.

PEPTIC ULCER DISEASE

Erosions or ulcers of the stomach lining or first portion of the small bowel (duodenum) are very common, particularly among young adults. Nausea, vomiting and abdominal pain may result. There is no reason not to run with ulcers. Some experimental evidence indicates that ulcers may actually improve with vigorous exercise such as running. However, weakness or severe abdominal pain may indicate complications requiring medical therapy. Blood in vomit or stool may indicate bleeding ulcers, an emergency requiring immediate medical care.

COLITIS

Inflammation of the small and large bowels is known as regional enteritis and ulcerative colitis, respectively. These diseases may cause severe abdominal pain, bloody diarrhea and other complications. Symptoms may be aggravated by increased muscular bowel contractions associated with running, so consult your physician about the advisability of continuing workouts.

ILEOSTOMY AND COLOSTOMY

Some individuals who undergo abdominal surgery require diversion of the bowel to the abdominal wall where a plastic bag collects intestinal contents. Following the recuperative period, most patients engage in completely normal activity, including vigorous physical exercise such as running. Ostomy clubs are very active in most cities, helping people who have had this operation return to a normal life-style.

ABDOMINAL PAIN

Pain arising from abdominal organs is not well localized. Our brain often perceives this pain as cramps or a vague burning sensation felt in the chest or in the abdominal muscles. Typical patterns of "referred pain" are illustrated in Figure 16-2. Severe, recurrent or persistent abdominal pain can be a sign of serious disease and should always be evaluated by a doctor.

Diseases of the gallbladder, esophagus, stomach and first part of the small intestine usually cause pain in the upper portion of the abdomen and are frequently felt in the mid-chest region resulting in dull gnawing or burning pain known as heartburn. Pain from these organs is frequently associated with nausea, vomiting and belching.

Disease of the small intestine is usually referred to the region around the umbilicus (belly button), while pain from the large bowel usually causes pain in the lower abdomen. Pain from intestinal disease is usually crampy and is sometimes associated with bloating, abdominal distention, gas and the urge to defecate.

Pain from appendicitis may begin in the region of the umbilicus but usually localizes to the right lower part of the abdomen.

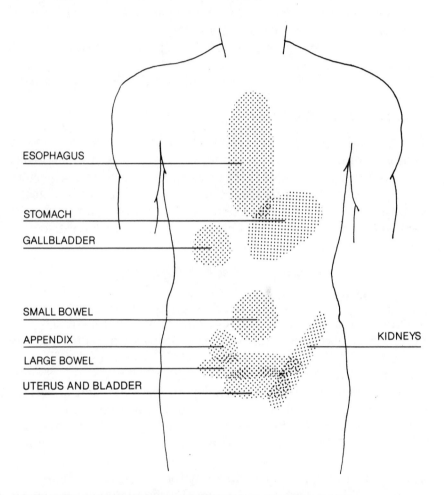

Pain from abdominal organs is not well localized. This figure illustrates common sites of discomfort or pain associated with diseases of the abdominal organs.

Figure 16-2.   REFERRED PAIN PATTERNS

Disease of the bladder, uterus or kidneys can cause pain in the groin, lower abdomen and pubic area.

Abdominal pain may also be associated with injury to the muscles of the abdominal wall such as pull or strain. This type of pain is usually sharp or pulling and is frequently aggravated by twisting or turning motions. Local tenderness of the abdomen is common.

17

Kidneys and Genitourinary System

Runners are often mistakenly informed that they have kidney disease. In reality, they are perfectly healthy, and the abnormal elements in their urine indicate "runners' kidneys," a minor ailment. Other runners, however, may damage their kidneys by improper training and racing schedules, particularly during hot weather.

Running can stimulate a runner's sex life. But runners should be aware of potential problems such as venereal disease, infertility, loss of periods and frostbite of the penis, occasionally associated with running.

URINARY TRACT

Basic Structure and Function

Blood is filtered by the kidneys at the rate of approximately 1200 cc* per minute. Water, electrolytes such as sodium and potassium, and metabolic waste products pass from the blood into the kidneys. Red blood cells and blood proteins do not usu-

* 1000 cc = 1 liter = 1.057 quarts

252

ally cross the kidney's filter. As the kidneys make urine, they also regulate the body's concentration of water, sodium, potassium, and acidity. Once urine is formed, it passes from the kidneys through long tubes (ureters) to the bladder where it is stored until urination via the urethra occurs (Figure 17-1).

Alterations During Exercise

During prolonged exercise, blood is shunted from the kidneys to the exercising muscle. The kidney partially compensates for this decreased renal (kidney) blood flow by becoming more efficient, allowing a greater percentage of the blood to be filtered. The overall result is that during prolonged exercise, the total urine output is decreased approximately 30 percent. The kidneys, however, can only partially compensate for water lost by sweating, making periodic water replacement absolutely necessary, especially during long runs. Conversely, the kidneys are very efficient at conserving salt (sodium), and deficiency of this element is rare. Potassium is frequently lost by the kidneys during exercise, resulting in low body potassium (see Chapter 18). The kidneys also excrete acids that build up in the body (hydrogen ions) during prolonged exercise.

Training the Kidneys

The kidneys undergo no specific adaptations with training. But training under hot conditions does lead to increased conservation of salt and water by the kidneys. As a result of increased body water, blood volume expands and a relative anemia occurs (Chapter 20).

Urinary Tract Problems

RUNNERS' KIDNEYS (ATHLETIC PSEUDONEPHRITIS)

Cause: Runners and other athletes often develop abnormal elements in the urine. Protein, red blood cells and clumps of red blood cells called casts are not normally found in urine, and their presence is usually a sign of a kidney disease called ne-

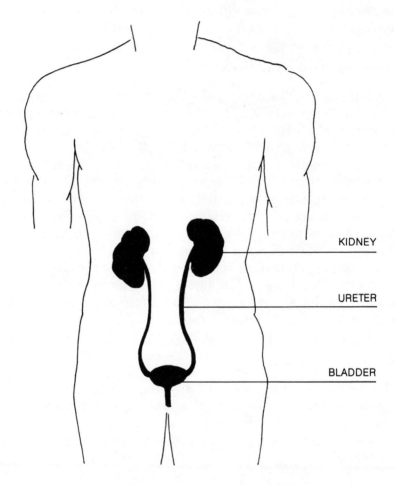

Urine is formed in kidneys, passes down ureters and is stored in bladder until urination.

Figure 17-1.   KIDNEYS AND URINARY TRACT

phritis. Healthy athletes may also have these abnormal elements present in the urine as a result of exercise. There are two basic mechanisms of athletic pseudonephritis. Individuals such as football players who engage in contact sports often have red blood cells in the urine as the result of trauma to the kidneys or the bladder. Runners, on the other hand, may have protein and casts in the urine. These abnormalities are thought to result from increased permeability of the kidney's normal filtering mechanisms associated with decreased blood flow to the kidneys during running. This condition is particularly common following long races and after hot weather running.

Symptoms and Diagnosis: Runners who develop pseudonephritis may notice dark urine, but there are usually no other symptoms. In contrast, people with true nephritis of the kidneys suffer from a variety of symptoms such as fatigue, nausea and water retention.

Most cases of athletic pseudonephritis are detected during routine physical examination and urine analysis. If a doctor is unaware of the patient's athletic status, kidney disease may be mistakenly suspected. Runners are not immune to kidney disease, and abnormal urine elements may represent either pseudonephritis or real disease. Urine abnormalities from pseudonephritis usually disappear within 2 days when running is stopped. If abnormalities persist beyond that point, see your doctor for urine analysis and possibly other diagnostic tests, including measurement of waste products in the blood (blood urea nitrogen and creatinine), X rays of the kidneys (intravenous pyelogram) and internal examination of the bladder with an instrument called a cystoscope. In addition, a kidney biopsy may be required in certain cases.

Comments and Treatment: Most authorities think that athletic pseudonephritis causes no harm. It is wise, however, to make sure that abnormal elements in the urine do disappear when running is stopped. Since real disease of the kidneys can result in severe complications, a complete evaluation by a kidney specialist is recommended when the diagnosis is in doubt.

KIDNEY FAILURE (ACUTE TUBULAR NECROSIS)

Cause: Renal tubule cells which make urine in the kidney are susceptible to damage from a variety of substances, sometimes resulting in a temporary type of kidney failure called acute tubular necrosis. Symptoms may develop immediately after running or 1–2 days later. Dark urine is noticed with either low urine volume or complete lack of urine output. When waste products build up in the blood, other symptoms such as nausea, vomiting, high blood pressure and even seizures or coma, develop. Runners can develop kidney failure by three separate mechanisms: hemoglobinuria, myoglobinuria and heatstroke.

1. *Hemoglobinuria* is the result of red blood cell destruction, occurring when you run on hard surfaces. Red blood cells are destroyed in the blood vessels of the foot, and hemoglobin, the red blood cell protein, is released. This hemoglobin is filtered from the blood by the kidneys where it can damage renal tubule cells, resulting in kidney failure. About 15 percent of runners will have some hemoglobinuria after completing a marathon. Some individuals are more susceptible to this problem and develop hemoglobinuria during shorter runs. A hard stomping gait may be one of the predisposing factors. Runners who develop hemoglobinuria will note dark-colored urine an hour or two after running, particularly after long runs on hard surfaces. Dehydration associated with hot weather running greatly increases the likelihood of kidney damage.

2. *Myoglobinuria* is the result of muscle damage. Severe prolonged exercise of skeletal muscle, particularly by untrained individuals, can result in the inflammation and destruction of muscle cells. These cells release muscle protein called myoglobin into the bloodstream 24–48 hours after exercise, and myoglobin, like hemoglobin, can damage kidney cells, resulting in kidney failure. Dehydration also increases the chances of this complication. Certain runners appear particularly susceptible to myoglobinuria. Sore muscles usually develop within the first 24 hours after exercise and dark urine on the second day. It is more common in older individuals, particularly during the first 2 weeks of training. This syndrome is called "exertional rhab-

domyolysis." Highly trained athletes may have mild myoglobinuria *immediately after* exercise, especially in hot weather, but do not usually develop kidney problems.

3. *Heatstroke* can cause dehydration, low blood pressure and very low blood flow to the kidneys. The kidney tubule cells are damaged by lack of oxygen, and kidney failure frequently develops. Heatstroke is a much more common cause of acute tubular necrosis than either hemoglobinuria or myoglobinuria.

The symptoms associated with heatstroke are described in Chapter 18. Runners who develop kidney failure following heatstroke usually have low blood pressure and low urine output when they first receive medical attention.

Symptoms and Diagnosis: Because the kidneys normally concentrate urine to conserve water lost during sweating, dark urine is frequently seen following long runs, particularly under hot conditions, and is usually harmless. But you should worry if you do not urinate within a few hours after a long run, particularly if you've had plenty to drink after the race or workout. Very dark urine (either red or cola colored) or persistent low urine volume should be brought to medical attention. The diagnosis of acute tubular necrosis can be made by analysis of blood and urine samples. Kidney failure is a serious condition which must be diagnosed and treated by medical experts.

Comments and Treatment: Fortunately, acute tubular necrosis is a reversible type of kidney failure since damaged tubule cells regenerate. However, since recovery may take up to 2 weeks, temporary measures are necessary to prevent complications. Runners who do develop kidney failure should be hospitalized under the care of a nephrologist (kidney specialist). Treatment may include dietary and fluid restrictions and the use of artificial kidneys to remove body wastes normally cleared by the kidneys.

Some unfortunate individuals who suffer kidney failure from acute tubular necrosis do not recover. A number of patients develop permanent kidney disease. In addition, the death rate associated with acute tubular necrosis is high even with good medical care. Therefore, proper precautions are strongly advised:

- *Adequate water replacement* during prolonged hot weather running is the single *most important* preventive measure.
- Individuals prone to hemoglobinuria should use foam rubber inner soles to cushion their feet.
- A sensible, *gradual* training program should prevent muscle damage from exertional rhabdomyolysis.

RUNNERS' HEMATURIA (BLOODY URINE)

Cause: Hematuria or blood in the urine must be distinguished from hemoglobinuria. In the case of hemoglobinuria, urine contains hemoglobin protein from red blood cell destruction. Hematuria means that intact red blood cells are present in the urine. Blood in the urine can result from disease that causes local bleeding at any point in the kidneys, ureters, bladder, or urethra. This long list includes kidney stones, tumors, infections, and many other conditions. Some runners, however, develop hematuria not associated with these usual disease processes. Authorities disagree as to the cause of runners' hematuria, and there are probably several different mechanisms. These include varieties of pseudonephritis already described, localized inflammation or bruises of the bladder and minor damage of veins at the outlet or neck of the bladder.

Symptoms and Diagnosis: Hematuria may be visible with the naked eye, in which case urine is dark or red in color. Milder cases of hematuria can be detected only when urine is examined through a microscope. Kidney stones can cause considerable pain in the flanks, groin and testicles. Burning on urination and fever usually result from urinary infections. On the other hand, runners' hematuria is painless and usually disappears within 2–3 days after cessation of running. But any runner who develops bloody urine should consult a physician to exclude other diseases. In addition to examining the urine, a doctor will probably evaluate the kidneys by X ray. Internal bladder examination with a cystoscope is also usually recommended. Only when all other possibilities are excluded should a diagnosis of runners' hematuria be made.

Comments and Treatment: True runners' hematuria appears to be a self-limited benign condition that does not require treatment. While some authorities have alternatively suggested running with full or empty bladders to prevent runners' hematuria, there appears to be no generally accepted treatment or preventive measure.

KIDNEY DAMAGE FROM LOW BODY POTASSIUM (SEE CHAPTER 18)

REPRODUCTIVE SYSTEM

Basic Structure and Function

MALE REPRODUCTIVE SYSTEM

Sperm develop in the testes and pass through a tube called the vas deferens to the urethra, where they are mixed with fluid from the prostate and other glands (Figure 17-2). The process of erection and ejaculation is controlled by nervous impulses. Testes also produce a male hormone called androgen (testosterone), which circulates throughout the body, causing male characteristics such as growth of facial hair, muscular development and a deep male voice.

FEMALE REPRODUCTIVE SYSTEM

The two ovaries contain human eggs (ovum) in various stages of development (Figure 17-3). Each month, midway between menses, a single ovum is discharged into a fallopian tube where it begins its passage to the uterus. If fertilization takes place in a fallopian tube, a fertilized egg implants on the uterus, resulting in a pregnancy. Female external genitalia (clitoris and labia) surround the vaginal canal which leads to the opening of the uterus (cervix). The monthly female cycle is regulated by two female hormones (estrogen and progesterone) that are secreted by the ovaries and controlled by the pituitary gland. Female sex characteristics, such as distribution of body fat and development of female breasts, are under control of these female hormones.

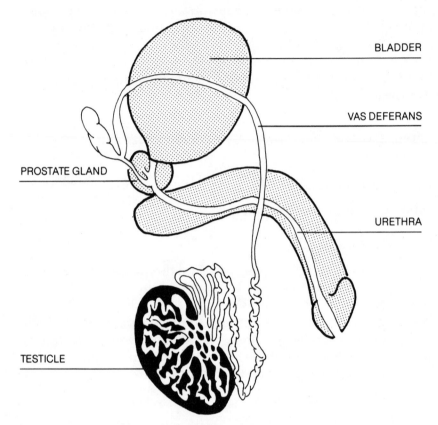

BLADDER

VAS DEFERANS

PROSTATE GLAND

URETHRA

TESTICLE

Figure 17-2.   MALE REPRODUCTIVE SYSTEM

Running and Sex

Many runners, both male and female, claim running increases the frequency and enjoyment of sexual activity. Needless to say, we runners are a slim and healthful lot, and we should expect to enjoy an active sexual life. In reality, some studies do indicate increased frequency and heightened enjoyment of sex among athletes in general. Authorities also report improved sex life among sedentary middle-aged men who pursue a regular exercise program, specifically a jogging rehabilitation program. But

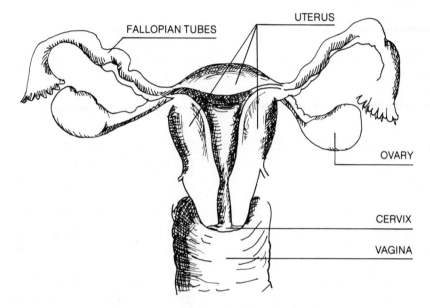

Figure 17-3. FEMALE REPRODUCTIVE SYSTEM

the infamous "runners keep it up longer" T-shirts must be considered folklore until more concrete scientific proof is available.

In contrast to increased sexual activity, there is some evidence that fertility may be adversely affected by running. This statement applies to both male and female runners. Low sperm counts have been demonstrated in male runners, and decreased menstruation or complete loss of periods (amenorrhea) is sometimes noted among women runners, particularly those with low body fat.

One of the drawbacks of a young runners' active sex life is an increased risk of venereal disease. Gonorrhea has reached epidemic proportions in the United States, and a runner's high state of physical fitness does not protect him or her from infection. Spread of gonorrhea is by oral or genital contact. Not all infected persons develop symptoms; a significant percentage of both men and women are asymptomatic carriers who can spread disease to sexual contacts. Gonorrhea can cause serious complications in both sexes, including sterility and spread of infection into the bloodstream. Since gonorrhea is readily cured with antibiotics such as penicillin, male runners who develop discharge or drip from the penis and females who note unusual vaginal discharge should seek medical help. In view of our current sexual standards, the only shame of gonorrhea is reluctance to obtain medical care.

Female Problems

MENSTRUATION

A Scandinavian study showed that young girls on a track team began menstruating approximately one year later than their non-running peers. Moreover, many women runners, especially those with low body fat, note irregular periods or complete loss of menses. It is probably not healthy for women to lose weight to such an extent that periods cease. Not only are they flirting with malnutirition, they may also be sacrificing endurance benefits thought to be associated with a higher percentage of body fat.

Women are divided as to whether menstruation affects their racing abilities, although careful studies reveal that objective performance is not impaired by menstruation. Menstruating females have won many gold medals at the Olympic games. Of course, there is considerable individual variation. Many women athletes subjectively feel weaker during this time. Serious competitors might wish to use birth control pills to prevent menses at the time of a particularly important race. The benefits of this practice, however, must be carefully balanced against recent studies that reveal severe side effects associated with the use of these drugs.

While most women claim that running decreases the pain of menstrual cramps, some have noted the opposite effect. Swedish investigators claim that training reduces menstrual cramps. Once again, individual variation is evident. Women who note severe menstrual cramps during running should either decrease their mileage or stop running completely for a few days. Since most people run for fun, there doesn't appear to be much sense in continuing with painful menstrual cramps. Resting a few days a month will certainly not impede the long range benefits of running. Each runner, therefore, must balance for herself the pleasure of running against the pain of menstrual cramps. Fluid retention often causes bloating and swelling of the legs (edema) for a few days before menses, and running usually helps these symptoms.

PREGNANCY

The majority of good women runners are able to run throughout most of their pregnancy. As long as a woman is accustomed to running, this exercise is probably beneficial during pregnancy. Certain situations, however, such as abnormal position of the placenta or weakness (incompetence) of the cervix can be aggravated by running. It is therefore important to consult an obstetrician early during a pregnancy to make certain that continued running is not dangerous.

INTRA UTERINE DEVICES (IUD)

IUDs are safe and effective methods of birth control that prevent implantation of fertilized eggs in the uterus. These foreign bodies occasionally cause uterine cramps, which in some women are aggravated by running. In most cases, however, women with IUDs experience no difficulty while running. If cramps persist, alternative methods of birth control are usually warranted.

BREASTS

Breasts are composed of fat and glandular tissues. The claim that running causes sagging of the breasts is untrue. Running with or without a bra will not damage the breasts, and to the contrary, many women develop firmer breasts from running. Wearing a bra is a matter of personal comfort, although a properly fitted bra with adequate support will generally be more comfortable for women runners with large breasts. Expect some reduction in breast size along with general decrease in body fat. Nipple abrasions are not as common a problem among women as they are among men. When necessary, petroleum jelly or Band Aids will prevent this problem.

Male Problems

POTENCY

The ability of men to engage in sexual intercourse is called potency. This function is controlled by a nervous reflex that governs erection and ejaculation. Running does not alter potency, although a runner's sexual drive is frequently increased, possibly as a result of increased energy and vigor. It is difficult to explain why many people claim that running prolongs sexual intercourse. The sexual act does not require high levels of aerobic or anaerobic fitness. Pulse rate does not usually exceed 120, well below aerobic capacity. Nevertheless, because of many personal communications, we will await scientific evidence before dismissing this claim.

FERTILITY

The ability to produce pregnancy is known as male fertility. There is no general trend regarding infertility among runners. Those runners, however, who are unable to cause pregnancy should be aware that running can cause low sperm counts. A couple should not worry about infertility until they have spent at least one year unsuccessfully trying to produce a pregnancy. Both partners should be evaluated. A male runner should consult either a urologist (male genitourinary specialist) or an endocrinologist (hormone and gland specialist).

PROSTATE DISEASE

Inflammation of the prostate gland is a common condition among middle-aged and older men and is often extremely uncomfortable. Unfortunately, the disease is not well understood. While running does not cause prostate disease, men who have it should be aware that dehydration may aggravate their symptoms, and they should be particularly careful to maintain adequate body hydration during and after running.

PENILE FROSTBITE

During cold weather jogging, the skin temperature of the penis can plummet to dangerous levels, resulting in frostbite symptoms. A running physician first noted and reported this ailment in an oft-quoted letter to the *New England Journal of Medicine*. The combination of cold and wind increase the danger of frostbite. Because nylon is a superior barrier to wind than cotton, cold weather runners should use nylon running shorts or warm-up pants, particularly during windy days. Cotton sweatshirts, shorts, and underwear are too porous to keep the skin warm during a stiff wind, but can be worn in layers with nylon shorts included. Unfortunate runners who develop numbness, tingling, or pain in the penis during cold weather runs should stop and warm the involved organ with the heat of the hands. Avoid vigorous rubbing which may injure the skin.

18

Hot Weather Problems

Hot weather is probably the single greatest hazard facing runners. With the exception of the automobile, running in hot weather is the quickest way to be killed. The adage to "know your body" is of special relevance to temperature regulation and water balance. Many misguided authorities think that runners can travel long distances without replacing fluids. While these same "experts" would never drive their automobiles without oil in the crankcase, they would force runners to run slowly out of body water and overheat in hot weather. On the assumption that these people are confusing the human body with the anatomy of camels, we call this group the "camel cult," and runners who adhere to their philosophy as possessors of a "camel complex."

Each year thousands of runners experience mild complications during hot weather running, while other less fortunate individuals develop severe disease and even die as a result of heat stress. Not only will an alert runner use this information to prevent illness, he will also use it to improve his running.

The human body has two closely related defenses against heat: temperature control (thermo-regulation), and salt and water regulation.

266

TEMPERATURE REGULATION

Basic Physiology

Body temperature normally fluctuates but slightly during the day. It is kept almost constant by a thermo-regulatory center in the brain, which continually monitors blood temperature. This center adjusts body functions to increase heat loss in hot environments and to conserve heat under cold conditions. Most exercise physiologists use degrees centigrade (C°), and the following guide supplies both:

Degrees Fahrenheit (F°)	Degrees Centigrade (C°)
98.6	37.0
100.4	38.0
102.2	39.0
104.0	40.0
105.8	41.0
107.6	42.0

The body gains heat from its own organs and from the environment. Body organs, particularly muscles, generate heat during normal metabolic processes. As metabolism increases during vigorous exercise such as running, the metabolic heat production also increases. When environmental temperatures are greater than body temperature, the body gains heat from the surrounding hot air. In addition, infrared heat from direct sunlight can raise skin temperature 1–2 C° by radiation.

When metabolic or environmental heat increases the body temperature, the thermo-regulatory center begins a cooling response. Veins in the skin dilate and blood is shunted to the body's surface, bringing heat with it. Skin blood flow increases from a resting level of 5 percent to a maximum of 20 percent of the total cardiac output. In this way, heat is brought to the surface of the skin and dissipated to the environment by radiation. In addition, a sweating response occurs, and body heat is lost by evaporation of sweat. Under hot conditions, sweating is the most important way that the body cools itself. One liter of sweat will,

when completely evaporated, lose approximately 580 kilocals*
of heat. During maximum heat stress, the sweating rate can increase from a resting level of ½ liter a day to between 2–3 liters
an hour.

At any given moment, body temperature reflects metabolic
heat production, environmental temperature, evaporative sweat
loss, and radiant heat from the body to the environment or vice
versa. In addition, environmental humidity and air movement
can affect body temperature. Since sweat evaporates slowly in
air already laden with water, high humidity reduces the effec-
tiveness of the body's cooling system, and during humid
weather, a runner must sweat more to dissipate heat. Wind cur-
rents help cool a runner by increasing evaporation and therefore
speeding heat loss.

The body has limited resources to keep itself cool during hot
humid conditions, and these resources are completely dependent upon sufficient body fluids. This is particularly true when
metabolic heat production from running compounds the problem. Since 1 liter of sweat weighs approximately 2¼ pounds, a
runner who loses 2–3 liters of sweat an hour will rapidly become
dehydrated. If fluid losses are not replaced, body cooling cannot
continue.

The body is much better equipped to respond to cold temperatures. Blood vessels in the skin are constricted to keep blood in
deep veins away from the skin, thereby minimizing radiant heat
loss. This insulating mechanism conserves heat, and the core
(deep body) temperature is maintained while skin temperature
falls. In fact, temperature in the body's extremities may be several degrees below the core temperature, and during exposure to
extreme cold, the fingers and toes are vulnerable to numbness
and frostbite. The body also responds to cold by increasing the
metabolic rate, a process known as shivering. Large muscle
groups contract against each other in purposeless movements
which increase metabolic heat production.

---

* One kilocal is the amount of heat required to warm one kilogram of water one degree
centigrade.

Alterations with Running

Running greatly increases the body's metabolic heat production. Body temperature increases in direct proportion to a work load as measured by a percentage of maximum oxygen uptake (Figure 18-1). Long distance runners increase their heat production 10–15 times over resting levels. Metabolic heat can approach 1,000 kilocals per hour. Body temperature quickly increases at the beginning of exercise. As temperature cooling mechanisms begin to operate, the body temperature usually levels off at 1–2 C° over resting values. During long runs in warm

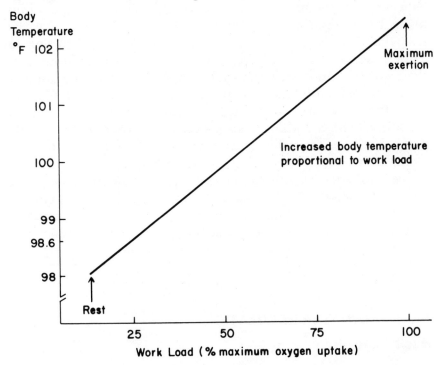

As work load (percent maximum oxygen uptake) increases, the body temperature increases as a result of metabolic heat production.

**Figure 18-1.   EXERCISE INCREASES
BODY TEMPERATURE**

weather, the body temperature frequently approaches dangerous levels. By the end of a marathon race, under mild environmental temperatures (70–80° F), deep muscle temperature approaches 106° F (41°C); rectal temperature usually ranges between 102–106° F (39–41°C).

As we know, the thermo-regulatory center tries to dissipate metabolic heat during running. Blood is shunted to the skin and sweating increases. In cool environments the body can easily dissipate metabolic heat by evaporative sweat loss alone. Under hot humid conditions, however, a dangerous situation soon develops because metabolic needs of the body compete with thermo-regulatory demands. There is competition for blood flow between exercising muscles and dilated skin vessels. Fluid losses from sweating soon aggravate this problem. As sweat is lost, the volume of blood in the circulation falls, resulting in extra stress on the heart. Blood pressure and stroke volume of the heart fall, and heart rate increases in order to maintain cardiac output. Finally, there is no extra fluid left in the circulation. Then the body must maintain blood pressure at the expense of sweating, which suddenly slows or stops completely. At this point, a runner is unable to dissipate his metabolic heat. Body temperature quickly skyrockets, causing heatstroke.

Even under less critical conditions, the heart must work harder in hot weather. For example, a runner's heart rate may be 120 while running a 6-minute mile at 60° F. When the temperatures reach 90° F, the same runner's heart rate may be 160 while he runs an identical 6-minute mile pace (Figure 18-2).

SALT AND WATER REGULATION
Basic Physiology

In the same way that the body maintains a relatively stable body temperature, it also tries to keep the total body water content relatively constant. Electrolytes are various salts dissolved in body fluids. These include sodium, potassium, magnesium, calcium, phosphorus and many minor elements. Each of these elements is essential for the normal functions of body cells. So-

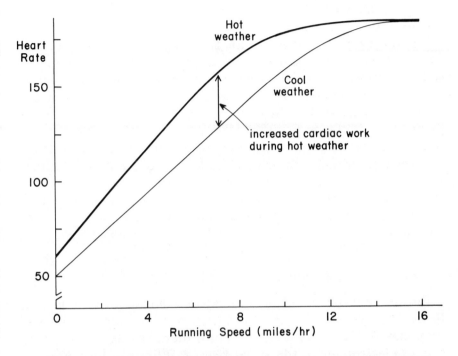

Heart must work harder because a large percentage of cardiac output is shunted to the skin to cool the body. Therefore, a runner's heart must work harder to maintain his race pace during hot weather.

Figure 18-2.   HEART RATE INCREASES DURING HOT WEATHER RUNNING

dium chloride, commonly known as salt, and potassium are the two electrolytes of special importance to runners.

In order to understand the physiology of body water and electrolytes, one needs only a simple balance sheet. Water is taken into the body in liquids and in food, and is also derived by metabolism of glucose. Water is lost by the body from the intestines, from the lungs as water vapor, from the skin as sweat, and from the kidneys as urine. When extra water is ingested, normal kidneys can easily increase urine output to keep the total body water content steady. To some extent, the kidneys can compensate for decreased water intake. Urine is concentrated and urine volume falls. But since some water is always lost from sources described above, dehydration will eventually result from prolonged water deprivation.

The electrolytes, sodium chloride and potassium, are normal constituents of the diet. Table salt is the most common source of sodium chloride, while potassium is present in many meats, fruits and vegetables. These electrolytes are lost from the body primarily in the urine. Sweat contains only small amounts of them.

When body stores of sodium are low, the kidneys are able to conserve it, reducing the danger of low body sodium chloride. Kidneys do not, however, conserve potassium, and loss continues even in the face of low body potassium, which therefore becomes a much greater potential danger than low body sodium chloride.

Alterations with Running

During running blood is shunted to exercising leg muscles. Blood flow to the kidneys decreases, and urine output falls approximately 30 percent. As sweating increases, the concentration of electrolytes in the sweat rises, resulting in loss of body sodium and potassium.

While the kidney does its best to conserve water and salt, the body's temperature control demands are much more important. Therefore, the result of prolonged exercise is loss of body water, sodium and potassium, especially in hot weather. Since sweating rates approach 2–3 liters an hour, loss of body water is almost always the most critical danger. There is still disagreement about the real significance of sodium and potassium losses during heavy exercise. While electrolyte loss is rarely an acute problem, chronic loss of these elements over a period of several days or weeks of hot weather running may cause problems.

Training Adaptations and Heat Acclimatization

After several days of running in hot climates, body changes occur that help maintain low body temperature during exercise. These changes are called heat acclimatization. The basic adaptations are: an increased sweating rate; an increase in blood water content or plasma volume, allowing extra reserve of fluid for sweating; an increased blood flow to skin in response to heat. The end result of heat acclimatization is the maintenance of a lower body temperature during running.

A runner must exercise in hot weather for approximately 2 weeks to achieve full heat acclimatization. But partial acclimatization occurs under other circumstances. Sedentary people living in hot climates are partially acclimated to heat. Training alone, even under cold weather conditions, causes partial heat acclimatization. A cold weather runner can further enhance his acclimatization by training while wearing extra clothing, such as a second sweatsuit. Physicians caring for the German national team claim that they are able to keep their athletes totally heat acclimated year round by having them take a steambath at 180° F for 20 minutes three times a week. Many runners in this country, particularly in the northeast, use one of these methods to achieve acclimatization during winter months prior to hot weather springtime races.

HOT WEATHER DISEASES

There are five basic complications that can develop from hot weather: chronic dehydration, low body potassium, heat cramps, heat exhaustion and heatstroke.

CHRONIC DEHYDRATION

Cause: The body's thirst mechanisms do not completely compensate for water lost in sweat during hot weather running. As a result, runners frequently do not drink enough fluids to replace sweat losses. A state of mild dehydration can develop producing a 1–3 percent body weight loss (1 quart of sweat weighs approximately 2¼ pounds). This process is usually insidious, developing over a period of several days.

Symptoms and Diagnosis: Chronic dehydration can cause generalized fatigue and listlessness. An avid runner may lose interest in his sport. Since 1 percent loss of body fluids will impair exercise performance, decreased running ability usually occurs. People suffering from chronic dehydration are very susceptible to more severe forms of heat-related diseases such as heatstroke. One of the most sensitive clues to total body water content is body weight. A runner who notes a sudden drop in body weight during hot weather should be alert to the possibility of chronic dehydration.

Comments and Treatment: Drink *at least* an extra quart of water daily during hot weather. If body weight suddenly falls, rest and drink enough water to regain normal weight. When symptoms of fatigue, listlessness and poor running form develop, take a few days off.

It is virtually impossible for a person with normal kidneys to drink too much water. When in doubt—*DRINK!*

LOW BODY POTASSIUM

Cause: Some authorities claim that low body potassium is relatively common, particularly during the first week of acclimatization. As we've stated, the kidneys do not conserve potassium well, and more is lost in urine and sweat than is replaced by diet. When the process of acclimatization is complete, body potassium usually returns to normal. Medical researchers don't agree about the incidence of potassium deficiency in runners. Some think that the problem is common, while others claim it is rare. However, some runners are prone to chronic low body potassium, particularly during hot weather running.

Symptoms and Diagnosis: Low body potassium can lead to mild damage of the kidneys and to generalized fatigue and muscle cramps. It also increases a runner's susceptibility to heatstroke. Increased urine volumes, particularly at night, may be a sign of kidney damage secondary to low body potassium. This disorder can be confirmed by analysis of blood potassium. Treatment should consist of increased intake of dietary potassium. Good food sources include citrus fruits, bananas, dates, raisins and meat. Avoid potassium supplements which are too concentrated, potentially dangerous and even fatal if used improperly. Potassium deficiency is usually a temporary process occurring during heat acclimatization, and it is best treated by decreased running and increased dietary intake of potassium.

HEAT CRAMPS

Cause: Heat cramps may result from acute sodium deficiency occurring during a strenuous workout under hot humid conditions. They usually develop in well-trained individuals who are already heat acclimated and who replace water but not enough salt lost in sweating. They may also be caused by a nervous reflex originating in a minor muscle tear or injury. Dehydration may increase this response. Whatever the mechanism, some people are prone to heat cramps.

Symptoms and Diagnosis: Heat cramps are brief intermittent muscle cramps, usually of the leg or abdominal muscles. They frequently occur after a workout, during a shower, or while asleep, although they may also develop at the end of a long workout or race. They can be very painful and disabling.

Comments and Treatment: This problem can sometimes be minimized by increasing sodium intake during hot weather exercise. Extra table salt with meals or two salt tablets taken prior to exercise are usually sufficient. Most individuals do not develop heat cramps and low body sodium is not usually present under hot weather conditions. The average American diet contains adequate salt for most runners. Since too much salt can sometimes cause high blood pressure, most runners shouldn't use salt tablets or large amounts of table salt.

HEAT EXHAUSTION

Cause: People who are not accustomed to exercise in hot environments can suffer heat exhaustion from loss of either water or salt. Symptoms usually develop when approximately 1–2 percent of body weight is lost.

Symptoms and Diagnosis: Heat exhaustion causes thirst, fatigue, generalized weakness, anxiety and impaired mental judgment. Severe cases can progress to hysteria, agitation, convulsions and coma. In most cases, dehydration is the predominant problem; sweating may be diminished and body temperature will rise. In rare cases, salt depletion is the major problem; sweating continues and there is usually no thirst. But nausea, vomiting, diarrhea, skeletal muscle cramps and low blood pressure associated with normal body temperature are noted.

Comments and Treatment: Runners who become extremely weak while running should immediately stop exercising, lie down in a cool spot, and, unless nauseated, drink plain water. Intravenous fluids are necessary in delirious or comatose people. Emergency salt replacement is rarely, if ever, necessary. If decreased sweating and increased body temperature are noted, the runner should be treated for heatstroke.

HEATSTROKE

Cause: Heatstroke is an extremely dangerous condition that usually occurs in people not accustomed to exercising in heat. But runners with chronic dehydration as well as persons with low potassium are also at increased risk as are older individuals with chronic heart disease. In addition, antihistamines may impair sweating and increase the likelihood of developing heatstroke. Failure to replace the water lost during prolonged exercise ultimately leads to decreased blood pressure, increased heart rate, decreased cardiac output and eventual fatigue of the sweat gland process. As a result, a runner is unable to dissipate metabolic heat, and body temperature rises very quickly to levels of 41° C (106°F) and above. Damage to the heart, kidneys, brain and liver results from high temperatures and low blood flow to these vital organs.

Symptoms and Diagnosis: In addition to body temperature greater than 106° F, heatstroke is characterized by changes in mental status such as delirium, aggressiveness, disorientation, seizures and coma. Cessation of sweating was once described as the third component of the triad of heatstroke symptoms. It is now apparent, however, that this symptom is more common in older nonrunners who are exposed to hot temperatures. Runners with heatstroke usually continue to sweat to some degree; their skin is not hot and dry.

Comments and Treatment: Heatstroke is a medical emergency. Race officials should have rectal thermometers available as part of routine equipment for hot weather races. Runners who develop impaired mental function or who collapse during hot conditions should have their body temperature measured immediately. A rectal temperature of 106° F or greater is diagnostic of heatstroke.

Remember that high body temperature is the most immediate threat to life; therefore a runner must be rapidly cooled by laying him down in a cool place, vigorously rubbing his body with ice and fanning him with cardboard to promote heat loss (some authorities recommend immersion in ice water baths). When his temperature falls to 102° F, discontinue cooling measures.

Once cooling has been started, water replacement should also begin. Because of low blood flow to the intestine, water taken by mouth may not get into the circulation for a long time. In addition, stuporous individuals may vomit and aspirate water into the lungs. For these reasons, fluid should be replaced intravenously and not by mouth.

Runners suffering from heatstroke should be rushed to the nearest hospital. Since complications from electrolyte imbalance may develop as well as heart, brain, kidney and liver damage, these unfortunate runners must be closely watched for several days.

To avoid this serious condition, take preventive measures. Replace water losses frequently. Only camels are designed to store water for long periods of time in desert climates. Humans are designed to drink frequently to replace body fluids lost in hot climates. Those distance runners who pretend they are camels are flirting with serious disease and possible death. Unfortunately, every once in a while, a nationally prominent runner will complete a marathon without drinking water. Other runners then try to emulate this example, thinking they can shave a few precious seconds from their running time. As a result serious complications occur. This absurd practice should logically be called a "camel complex" and should be categorized with the "superman complex" and other assorted death wishes that occasionally give distance running a bad name. Runners continue to die each year from heatstroke. A runner should never run in hot weather without frequent water stops. Coaches and race officials who advise otherwise are wrong. These members of the antiquated "camel cult" are apparently unaware of how the human body keeps itself cool.

Despite the urging of medical authorities, race officials continue to hold long distance events during hot, humid weather. Maximum sweating probably occurs at 68° F, and therefore, a runner's temperature must increase when race day temperatures exceed 68° F. Additional factors that increase body temperature are relative humidity and radiant heat. For this reason, the wet bulb globe temperature index (WBGT) was devised. Temperatures are recorded from: a standard thermometer in the shade; a black glove thermometer in the sun and wind; a standard wet bulb thermometer also placed in the sun and wind. The WBGT is calculated by adding $\frac{7}{10}$ of the wet bulb reading, $\frac{2}{10}$ of the black globe, and $\frac{1}{10}$ of the standard thermometer in the shade. When the WBGT exceeds 28° C (82.4° F), long distance races greater than 10 kilometers should be canceled. Unfortunately this advice remains unheeded. In 1976 sixteen runners were hospitalized for heat-related diseases following the Boston Marathon. In 1978 three runners died during a Japanese marathon held under unfavorable environmental conditions. A world class runner almost died from heatstroke during the famous Falmouth race, less than 8 miles long.

During borderline weather conditions, the danger can be minimized or avoided if proper precautions are taken. Runners who have symptoms suggestive of chronic dehydration or low body potassium should definitely not compete until these conditions are corrected. A runner who develops heat exhaustion or heatstroke should never again compete under hot conditions, as there is an increased risk of a second attack.

Remember that intestinal absorption may lag behind oral ingestion, and start drinking before the start of a long distance race. During the race, take every opportunity to drink plain water. Since a trained runner can lose between 2–3 liters of sweat an hour, he should try to replace fluids accordingly—at least 8–10 ounces every 15 minutes. (See Chaper 16 for further discussion of fluid ingestion during running.)

A racing jersey covers approximately 30 percent of the body's surface. Since this material interferes with sweat evaporation, many runners prefer to race without a shirt during hot, humid conditions. Generally speaking, this practice is sound and will facilitate loss of body heat. Under extreme environmental temperatures, however, light-colored or reflecting clothing will protect against the radiant heat of the sun. AAU rules state that a runner must wear a shirt. Check with race officials before an event to find out if they plan to enforce this regulation, or wear a fishnet jersey which will meet the requirement and still allow evaporation of sweat.

During hot weather training or racing, set realistic goals. Long distance racing records are never set during very hot conditions, and it is foolish to push for a personal best in extreme heat. During training runs, a sensible practice is to use pulse rate rather than speed as a measure of intensity of the workout. Most important, don't fall victim to the camel cult. Remember that water is necessary to cool the human body. If you can't drink, don't run.

19

Diabetes and Hypoglycemia

Two percent of Americans have diabetes, and the incidence of this disease is increasing. Running is a natural sport for diabetics. It often helps control the disease and may even prevent some of the terrible complications. Moreover, running may prevent diabetes altogether in some individuals with an inherited tendency to this disease. However, diabetic runners must take special precautions to avoid low blood sugar shock and skin infections.

Diabetes Mellitus

Cause: Diabetes is a common disease characterized by abnormality of fat and carbohydrate metabolism. Insulin, a protein enzyme made by the pancreas, plays a major role in the uptake of blood sugar (glucose) by the body's cells. On a simplified level, people with diabetes do not produce adequate insulin to metabolize properly the carbohydrates needed for the body's daily functions. As a result, blood sugar increases and abnormalities in fat metabolism occur. Symptoms vary from mild blood sugar elevation to severe illness with disease of the heart and blood vessels, the nervous system and the kidneys. Tendency to develop diabetes is frequently inherited, but obesity increases both the chances of developing diabetes and the overall severity of the disease.

Vigorous exercise such as running is of special importance to diabetics and to people with a family history of diabetes. Many experts think that regular exercise facilitates control of the disease and prevents long-term complications. In addition, many people with strong family histories of the disease have either a mild case of diabetes or a tendency towards diabetes called "latent diabetes" or "prediabetic state." Evidence indicates that proper diet and exercise therapy may alter the chances of developing diabetes and diabetic complications among these susceptible people.

Symptoms and Diagnosis: Juvenile diabetes, which is acquired at a young age, is usually more severe than adult-onset diabetes, which occurs during middle life. Young diabetics frequently develop very high blood sugars associated with fatigue, weight loss, increased appetite and frequent urination. Sugar in the urine draws water out of the body, causing dehydration and thirst. Severe cases may result in extreme abnormalities of body water and electrolyte balance, high blood acid and even coma and death. Diabetics have an increased tendency to develop infection, particularly skin infections, which are often resistant to normal healing. With time, diabetics develop premature coronary artery disease, atherosclerosis, chronic kidney disease, stroke, peripheral nerve disorders, cataracts, and disease of the retina of the eyes. While some studies indicate decreased strength and endurance among juvenile diabetics, many of these children are able to perform competitively in sports.

The majority of adults with mild diabetes and those with prediabetic state have no symptoms, and diabetes often goes undetected for several years. It is during this latent period that silent damage to blood vessels occurs, finally culminating in premature atherosclerosis and many of the other complications of diabetes.

Diabetes can usually be diagnosed by simple measurement of blood sugar. This test is performed in the morning before breakfast and again after a high carbohydrate meal. Analysis of blood sugar usually reveals both overt diabetes and prediabetic state. People with diabetes have a high fasting blood sugar and an abnormal rise after carbohydrate ingestion. Prediabetic individuals may have only a mild elevation of fasting blood sugar with an abnormal rise or fall after a carbohydrate meal (Figure 19-1).

Comments and Treatment: There are basically three types of treatment for diabetes: dietary changes to alter the pattern of carbohydrate and fat intake and to reduce weight; insulin injections or oral medication to increase pancreatic production of insulin; regular exercise to burn excess blood sugar.

Many famous athletes, both past and present, have suffered from diabetes. This disease should not discourage a young run-

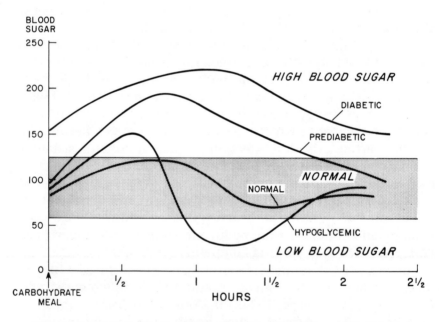

Diabetics have high fasting blood sugar which increases after meal. Prediabetic persons may have normal fasting blood sugar with abnormal rise after meal. Persons who develop hypoglycemic symptoms will have blood sugar fall below normal range approximately 45 to 90 minutes after a meal.

Figure 19-1.   BLOOD SUGAR AFTER CARBOHYDRATE MEAL (GLUCOSE TOLERANCE TEST)

ner from continuing his chosen sport. A proper combination of insulin and running usually facilitates control of blood sugar. Since vigorous exercise requires sugar for muscle metabolism, diabetics must make appropriate adjustments in their insulin dosage and dietary carbohydrate intake to compensate for sugar burned by running. The alteration of insulin dosage varies from individual to individual and must be methodically derived on the basis of careful experimentation under the supervision of a physician. Diabetic runners should generally run approximately the same amount each day in order to avoid drastic swings in blood sugar. Avoidance of insulin shock or low blood sugar hypoglycemia is absolutely essential. Diabetic runners can develop this complication when they run farther than normal without decreasing insulin dosage or increasing carbohydrate intake. Most diabetic athletes carry sugar cubes or some other readily available source of carbohydrate at all times in case of hypoglycemia symptoms, and all wear medical alert tags identifying them as diabetic. Diabetic runners should inject insulin in the abdominal wall rather than the thigh as the muscular action of running may speed absorption of insulin from the thigh and cause insulin shock. Diabetic runners must never run long distances alone and should make sure that their running partners know what to do if hypoglycemic symptoms strike.

The serious runner who has diabetes should carefully note alterations in insulin dosage and carbohydrate intake in his running diary. This is particularly important when calculating insulin and diet before long distance races such as marathons. Those who wish to compete in these events should carefully calculate the right combination during practice runs in excess of 20 miles. Diabetics are particularly susceptible to dehydration and accumulation of blood acid. They should be especially careful to drink adequate water during long distance races but must be cautious with drinks containing sugar, taking only small but frequent amounts to avoid drastic swings in blood sugar and "rebound hypoglycemia." Diabetics should identify themselves to officials before a race, in the event that difficulties develop.

Authorities used to recommend that diabetics structure diets to receive approximately 40 percent of calories from carbohydrate, 40 percent from fat, and 20 percent from high quality protein foods. Recent studies, however, indicate that the percentage of carbohydrate can be increased considerably, probably to the level of 70 percent, as long as the carbohydrate is of high quality (fruits, vegetables, complex sugars). Distance runners usually consume a much higher percentage of carbohydrate in the diet than do nonrunners. There seems to be no reason that diabetics need to alter this pattern as long as the carbohydrate is derived from quality food sources such as fruits and vegetables rather than from sweets and starches.

Diabetics are particularly susceptible to skin infections. Runners frequently develop blisters and small abrasions of the feet and legs. Diabetics must take meticulous care to avoid the development of serious skin infections complicating these minor injuries. Small cuts and abrasions should be carefully cleaned and covered, and running should be discontinued until blisters and abrasions of the feet are healed. Medical attention should be sought at the first sign of infection. Correctly fitting shoes are essential to all runners and an absolute must for diabetics. Feet should be carefully washed, dried and powdered after each workout. In addition, pay particular attention to proper toenail cutting (Chapter 5) to avoid ingrown toenails and infections.

Many individuals with mild diabetes, particularly when it is acquired during middle age, can be treated with dietary restriction and weight loss. A high percentage of these people probably would be free of diabetes if they adopted a runner's life-style of diet, weight control and routine exercise. This category of diabetics should discuss such a program with their physicians.

Hypoglycemia

Low blood sugar is called hypoglycemia. As a rule, this is one of the most overdiagnosed disesases, particularly among neurotics. In reality, the regular development of low blood sugar is relatively unusual. Some cases are caused by the prediabetic state, while others are associated with insulin-producing tumors.

Many normal people, however, will occasionally develop mild hypoglycemia by fasting or during vigorous exercise. It most frequently occurs 45–90 minutes after a high carbohydrate meal when the body appears to overreact to the large sugar load, producing too much insulin. As a result, blood sugar falls (Figure 19-1). This is called the "rebound phenomenon," and some individuals do appear prone to this complication. Symptoms include: headache, dizziness, nausea, general weakness and sweating associated with a rapid pulse and pounding heart.

Some runners develop rebound hypoglycemia after eating carbohydrates 45 minutes to an hour before a race. Authorities, therefore, suggest that no sugar be taken during the hour before running. The magnitude of this problem is uncertain since running long distances usually has very little effect on blood sugar. Ultramarathon runners, however, do note hypogylcemia after 20–30 miles.

Those runners who occasionally note symptoms suggestive of hypoglycemia should confirm the diagnosis by analysis of blood sugar. Eating sugar usually rapidly reverses symptoms, and susceptible runners should carry sugar cubes. Avoiding large swings in blood sugar by spreading out dietary carbohydrate throughout the day will generally diminish the chances of developing hypoglycemia.

Other Endocrine Glands

The other endocrine glands of the body include the thyroid gland in the neck, which controls the overall rate of body metabolism; the parathyroid glands situated within the thyroid gland, which are responsible for calcium metabolism; the adrenal glands on top of the kidneys, which produce cortisone and adrenalin, substances necessary for many aspects of body metabolism; and the pituitary gland located in the brain, which secretes a variety of substances and orchestrates the function of the rest of the endocrine gland secretions. While these are undoubtedly important for maintaining body metabolism, they are not of special relevance to runners.

Generally speaking, runners with diseases of the endorcrine glands can safely continue running. This advice, however, should be confirmed by a physician.

20

Miscellaneous Problems

Runners frequently develop miscellaneous problems, including: headache, anemia, swollen glands and insect sting allergy.

Anemia (low blood count)

Cause: Red blood cells carry oxygen from the lungs to body tissues. These cells are composed primarily of hemoglobin, a protein with a strong affinity for oxygen, and are manufactured in the inner cavity of bones, the bone marrow. They enter the body's circulation and have an average life span of 120 days. Old blood cells are removed from the blood by the spleen and other organs, while the bone marrow constantly resupplies new red blood cells. When the blood count drops as a result of bleeding, the bone marrow is able to respond by producing more new cells. Moreover, under conditions of low oxygen such as high altitude, the bone marrow is stimulated to produce higher than normal numbers of red blood cells.

Anemia develops in several ways. Deficiency of iron, folic acid, or B_{12}, substances that are building blocks for red blood cells, will cause anemia. Chronic blood loss from ulcers or tumors in the gastrointestinal tract can eventually lead to anemia.

Chronic diseases such as infections and kidney failure often depress the bone marrow's normal production of red blood cells.

Many endurance athletes—swimmers, runners and Olympic athletes—suffer from anemia. Among its causes are: destruction of red blood cells in blood vessels of the feet (Chapter 17); loss of iron in sweat; decreased dietary intake of iron among some athletes who engage in fad diets that don't contain meat or iron-containing fruits or vegetables. Women lose blood during menstruation and are therefore more likely to be iron deficient and anemic. On the basis of studies of athletes, we can estimate that between 2–5 percent of runners suffer from mild anemia. One of the training effects previously mentioned is expansion of the blood volume. The fluid content of the blood increases when the body stores a little extra water as a safety margin for sweating. As a result of increased fluid in the blood, the red blood cell concentration is diluted, causing a falsely low blood count. This condition should be called "runners' pseudoanemia."

Symptoms and Diagnosis: Most individuals with mild anemia suffer no ill effects and have no symptoms. More severe loss of red blood cell oxygen-carrying capacity causes weakness and dizziness, particularly during vigorous exertion.

Blood count is easily measured with a small blood sample as part of a routine physical examination. In addition, blood iron, folic acid and B_{12} can be analyzed. Runners who are found to be anemic should be evaluated prior to treatment. Minimum evaluation includes analysis of stools for blood to uncover an unsuspected gastrointestinal ulcer or tumor. If there is no blood in their stools, it is reasonable to treat anemic menstruating females with iron supplements. Anemic men, however, and women past menopause should be more completely evaluated. Tests include X rays of the gastrointestinal tract and analysis of a small sample of bone marrow obtained with a needle.

Comments and Treatment: Maintenance of normal red blood cell count is important for maximum oxygen-carrying capacity. In fact, some athletes think that elevation of blood count will improve performance. This is the theory behind altitude training and the practice of blood doping by which stored red blood cells are transfused into an athlete just prior to competition. Blood doping is illegal under rules of international competition.

Iron, folic acid or B_{12} supplements offer no benefits to individuals who are not anemic. Although modest doses of these substances are not harmful, there is no reason to take them on a routine basis. While some authorities recommend iron supplements for women of childbearing age, this practice is probably unnecessary unless anemia is present.

Arthritis

Arthritis is inflammation of the joints. Basically, there are two broad categories of arthritis: degenerative (see Chapter 4) and inflammatory.

Degenerative arthritis represents a wear-and-tear process that is present to some extent in every individual over the age of twenty. Inflammatory arthritis is often a more serious and disabling disease. Types of inflammatory arthritis include: rheumatoid arthritis, gout and systemic lupus erythematosus. Many people mistakenly think that running will produce degenerative arthritis. To the contrary, studies indicate runners have a lower than normal rate of degenerative arthritis. Moreover, running often improves symptoms of degenerative arthritis. Runners with mild disease should therefore not be discouraged from running. It is wise, however, for these individuals to choose soft running surfaces to minimize the stress on their joints. Because running lowers the body's uric acid—the substance responsible for gout—it may actually offer some protection against this disease. There is no relationship between other types of inflammatory arthritis and running.

Individuals who suffer from these diseases generally should not run when acute flares of disease are present. When arthritis is medically controlled, running may offer some benefit for the maintenance of muscle strength and joint stability, but first should be discussed with a physician.

Cancer

Cancer is an abnormal growth of body cells which can invade and destroy normal tissue. There are many factors that cause it, including viruses, chemicals, toxins, and inherited susceptibility.

The relationship between athletics and cancer is debated. Some studies indicate higher cancer rates among athletes, while others reach the opposite conclusion. These conflicting results indicate need for further research. But some interesting studies deserve mention.

A few epidemiologic studies of athletes indicate a higher death rate from cancer, although the difference is statistically small. The significance of these findings is uncertain. Cancer, heart disease and accidents are the most common causes of death in the United States. Since athletes have lower death rates from heart disease, it naturally follows that they must eventually die from another cause. Therefore, it is not surprising that athletes may have a higher death rate from cancer, as well as from accidents.

In contrast, other studies indicate the opposite—a lower death from cancer among athletes. These findings may reflect "protective" dietary habits of athletes. Dietary animal fat is closely linked with bowel cancer. Vegetarians and other runners who avoid animal fat may be protected from bowel cancer.

Animal studies also indicate that vigorous exercise has protective value against cancer. Mice who have an inherited tendency to develop cancer exhibit a lower incidence of this disease when they are exercised daily. Another experiment with a strain of mice that develops breast cancer showed that body weight reduction very significantly decreased the occurrence of this tumor. Both of these studies would indicate, therefore, that runners' exercise and dietary habits offer some protection against cancer.

Of particular importance is the relationship between cigarette smoking and cancer. The fact that runners do not smoke certainly offers protection against lung cancer. This disease is one of the leading causes of death among cigarette smokers and is extremely rare among nonsmokers.

It should be emphasized that runners are not immune to cancer. The presence of a cardinal warning sign should immediately be brought to medical attention. These signs are:
1. The development of an abnormal swelling or lump
2. Unusual weight loss

3. The presence of blood in the stool

4. Chronic fever or fatigue

Those runners who do develop cancer need not give up running. Many types of cancer are either completely curable or well controlled by surgery, radiation and /or drug therapy (chemotherapy). Once the disease is controlled, there should be no reason to stop running. In one interesting study, in fact, running was part of the treatment for individuals with far advanced cancer. Although there was no effect upon the tumor, these patients frequently enjoyed psychological benefits from the running programs. Of course, each runner should discuss his training program with his physician to decide what is best for him.

Eye Problems

CONTACT LENSES

Over the past decade, technological advancements have resulted in lightweight comfortable contact lenses that can be worn from 12–18 hours a day. These devices offer many advantages. Contact lenses guarantee clear vision despite mud, rain, fog and other types of inclement weather. While eyeglasses are certainly adequate for most types of running, competitive runners, particularly cross-country racers, may wish to consider contact lenses.

BLIND RUNNERS

Several blind individuals have achieved admirable success at long distance running. The psychological benefits of this practice are obvious. Runners may wish to encourage blind friends to consider running.

Runners' Headache

Cause: There are several diseases that cause headache. These include: allergies; infections; diseases of the eyes, ears, nose, throat and teeth; inflammation of blood vessels and arthritis of the neck and the jaw; fever; high blood pressure; fatigue, tension and many general disease states. Moreover, some individuals develop recurrent headaches called migraine. All of these diseases usually cause headaches by one of two mechanisms: dilation of blood vessels that supply the brain, or spasms of scalp muscles.

While runners may develop headache from any of the above diseases, there is also a condition known as "effort headache" to which some runners are susceptible. Symptoms usually occur after strenuous workouts or races. Buildup of lactic acid and low blood carbon dioxide probably cause dilation of blood vessels supplying the brain, resulting in swelling of the brain and headache. Other factors predisposing to effort headache include hot weather, increased humidity, lack of training and high altitude. In addition, some authorities think that effort headaches are more common when a runner eats certain foods that cause dilation of blood vessels. These foods include cheeses, chocolates and alcoholic beverages.

Symptoms and Diagnosis: Effort headaches usually occur within an hour after a vigorous workout. Some unfortunate runners develop symptoms every time they run. The pain is usually in the front of the head, and there may be nausea, weakness, and vomiting.

Migraine headaches are a chronic problem that recur over a period of years. The symptoms vary considerably. Most typically, the pain is on one side of the head. Flashing light or strong smells may precede the headache. Extreme weakness, nausea, and vomiting are common.

Headaches due to high blood pressure, particularly upon rising in the morning, are typically located in the back of the head.

Sinus headaches are often aggravated by running. In this instance, fullness and pain is noted in the frontal sinuses above the eyes and the maxillary sinuses under the cheekbones. These symptoms are usually worse when the head is lowered. Fever and sinus discharge indicate infection (see Chapter 14).

Allergic headaches from pollens most often occur in the spring or fall months. Itchy eyes and sneezing are usual.

Pinpointing the cause of a headache is an extremely difficult and complicated medical problem. Runners who develop what appears to be effort headaches should discuss their symptoms with a physician. Any type of recurring headache should be thoroughly evaluated in order to exclude more serious disease. Tests include X rays of the skull, radioactive brain scans, and brain wave analysis (EEG).

Comments and Treatment: There is no clear agreement as to the best way to treat effort headache. The following precautions might be helpful: Avoid severe dehydration during running. Do not eat foods such as cheese, chocolate and alcoholic beverages for at least an hour after a run. High carbohydrate meals prior to running may be protective. Cold drinks often lend temporary relief. Diuretics or water pills remove excess body water and relieve brain swelling, thereby helping some cases.

Antihistamines usually help prevent sinus headaches. More complicated problems such as migraine should be evaluated by a neurologist (nervous system specialist).

Runners' Stroke

When blood flow to the brain is blocked, serious dysfunction of the nervous system soon develops. These symptoms include local weakness of the arms and legs, inability to speak, memory difficulties and many other problems. A few hapless runners have developed temporary and even permanent strokes. These complications may have been due to intense spasm of brain blood vessels, occurring within an hour after running. Some authorities claim that foods which stimulate blood vessel contraction and relaxation may cause this problem, as well as runner's headache. For this reason, a runner should be cautioned against eating cheeses, chocolates and alcoholic beverages within an hour after running. Runners who develop dizziness, difficulty speaking or weakness of an extremity should be rushed to the nearest hospital.

Running and Mental Illness

Several psychiatrists have noted that running is excellent therapy for depression. While application of this observation is still experimental, some severely psychotic patients have improved from running therapy. The greatest potential benefit appears to be in the area of mild depression. Running helps people relax and shed superficial tensions and anxiety. Many runners are able to relieve tension and solve personal problems while running.

Running addiction deserves mention. Many individuals note that running produces side effects similar to addicting medications. Runners frequently develop a compulsion to run, requiring more and more mileage to gain inner satisfaction. Withdrawal symptoms such as anxiety, irritability and mild headache occur if a runner is forced to lay off for a few days. Authorities refer to this type of dependence as positive addiction. This means that running is a healthy addiction as opposed to negative addictions such as alcoholism or narcotic abuse. Despite the positive aspects of running addiction, runners should not allow this sport to interfere with life's other essential activities. Like alcoholics and drug addicts, running addicts occasionally note that their compulsion is so strong it interferes with their work or family life. One of the best ways to prevent this type of obsession is to set clear-cut, realistic running goals. Runners should aim for particular races or seasons. In this way, an individual can work hard for a few weeks or months of the year, peaking for a special event, then curtailing the intensity of his running schedule for a rest period during which he catches up on other important aspects of his life.

Stinging Insect Allergy

Cause: Every year a large number of people in the United States die from allergy to insect stings. Runners are particularly vulnerable to this catastrophe because they spend time bounding through grassy fields and woods with bare limbs. Unfortunately, most individuals are unaware that they are allergic to insects until they are stung. Venom of bees, wasps or hornets may cause severe allergic reaction. Yellow jackets are the most common culprit.

Symptoms and Diagnosis: Severe allergic reactions often strike a perfectly healthy person. Symptoms begin within 15 minutes after a sting. Death may be so quick that it is attributed to heart attack. Other people are warned by swelling of a whole extremity, dizziness, wheezing, fainting, and shock after an insect sting. A runner who develops one of these reactions is likely to experience a more serious problem with the next sting, and he should see an allergist. Careful history and skin tests will confirm the diagnosis.

Comments and Treatment: There are three things that can kill a trained distance runner during a run: automobiles, heatstroke and an allergic reaction to an insect sting. Heart attacks are extremely rare in trained distance runners. Most likely some of those runners who die suddenly during a run are misdiagnosed as heart attack instead of insect sting allergy.

If a runner is stung, he should immediately stop running because continued exercise may aggravate an allergic reaction. If unusual symptoms occur, apply a tourniquet to the extremity above the sting, and place ice on the local site. If a runner becomes unconscious after a sting, give mouth-to-mouth resuscitation and adrenalin, if available. Immediate medical attention can be life saving.

If a runner has an allergic reaction to an insect sting, he should definitely see an allergist for shots to desensitize or make him less allergic. He will also be given a kit containing a syringe with adrenalin to carry with him in case of another sting and will be instructed in its use.

While many runners worry about snakes in the woods, insect stings are a much more dangerous possibility. People who exercise outdoors during the summer months are at risk. There is no doubt that many people reading this book would be in serious trouble if they were stung by a bee. A runner with insect allergy should always carry the emergency kit during out-of-door runs. A coach or trainer would be wise to have one available during outdoor practice. It may be life saving. On two occasions, I have seen people suddenly collapse following a bee sting—one on a tennis court and one on a golf course. Both would have died if they had not received adrenalin immediately.

Swollen Glands (lymphadenopathy)

Cause: Lymph glands are an important part of the body's defenses against infection. These organs are collections of white blood cells called lymphocytes. They filter bacteria and foreign particles that invade the body. Lymph glands are located throughout the body, but are concentrated in the neck, the underarms and in the groin. Swelling of lymph glands is called lymphadenopathy and can result from a variety of diseases such as infection and tumor. For example, infection in the mouth or throat can cause swelling of the lymph glands in the neck, while infection of the foot can lead to lymphadenopathy in the groin. Lymphadenopathy is a normal reaction to local inflammation as the lymph nodes fight invading bacteria. Generalized viral infections can cause swelling of lymph glands throughout the body. Tumors such as Hodgkin's disease and lymphoma involve lymph glands, causing local or generalized lymphadenopathy.

Runners frequently develop lymphadenopathy in the groin from repeated minor injuries of the feet. Small abrasions or blisters as well as fungal infections may be noticed. In many instances, however, the runner is completely unaware of the injuries to the feet.

Symptoms and Diagnosis: Lymphadenopathy is usually painless, but there is occasional tenderness, especially when lymph gland swelling occurs quickly. Fever suggests an infectious cause. The development of lymphadenopathy throughout the body, especially when associated with weight loss and fatigue, can indicate a more serious problem such as a tumor.

Most runners have small lymph glands in the groin, and one side is usually larger than the other. This condition is almost always a normal reaction to running and should cause no alarm. The location of lymphadenopathy generally helps pinpoint the problem. Infections of the mouth, the throat, the sinuses and the scalp cause swelling of the lymph glands in the neck. Swelling of glands above the clavicles usually represents tumor. Insect bites of the scalp and ringworm, a fungal scalp infection, cause swelling of glands in front of the ear, while German measles causes swelling behind the ear. Manual laborers and individuals who develop repeated trivial infections of the arms and hands often have lymphadenopathy around the elbow or under the arm.

Comments and Treatment: The runner should not be duly concerned about lymphadenopathy in the groin. More generalized involvement should always be brought to the attention of a physician. There is a myth that hard training alone can lead to generalized lymphadenopathy. Hard training may lead to increased susceptibility of infections (discussed in Chapter 13) which, in turn, may lead to inflammation of lymph glands.

Appendix

Runners' Medical Profile and Physicians' Reference

Trained runners differ from sedentary "normal" persons in several respects. These "abnormalities" actually reflect training adaptations and dietary preferences of runners. The average American is a sickly being with a body that ages prematurely from nicotine poisoning, overeating and lack of activity. Definitions of normal should be revised, therefore, defining the human body as it should be, not as it all too frequently is.

Nevertheless, runners often have difficulties obtaining life insurance and passing routine physical examinations. Physicians and other health personnel are frequently not aware that laboratory tests outside the normal range do not necessarily indicate disease in runners. Therefore, we provide a table of common deviations from normals found in runners and a brief comment explaining these abnormalities. Runners may wish to bring this information to their doctor's attention.

Common Deviation from Normal	Comment
PHYSICAL EXAMINATION:	
Bradycardia (slow heart)	Training effect, increased vagal tone, increased stroke volume
Hypotension (low blood pressure)	Training effect, usually 5–15 millimeters less than normal range
Lean Body Composition—low weight, high body density, low percent body fat	Result of training and diet; male runners less than 10 percent, female runners less than 18 percent body fat
Heart—hyperdynamic precordium, functional systolic murmur, loud S3	Increased stroke volume, increased left ventricular end diastolic volume
CHEST X RAY:	
Increased cardiac/thoracic Ratio	Left ventricular and right atrial hypertrophy commonly found; normal training adaptation
URINE ANALYSIS:	
Albuminuria, hematuria, protein casts	Athletic pseudonephritis (Chapter 17)
Ketonuria	Mild dehydration common
CBC:	
Decreased hematocrit—normal hemoglobin	Increased blood volume, iron deficiency anemia common (Chapter 20)
Increased white blood cell count, increased platelet count	Due to exercise stress, usually disappears a few hours after exercise
BLOOD LIPIDS:	
Decreased cholesterol, increased high-density lipoproteins, decreased low-density lipoproteins,	Result of diet, low percent body fat, and fatty acid metabolism during running—protective profile against coro-

Common Deviation from Normal	**Comment**
decreased very low-density lipoproteins, decreased triglycerides, increased high-density lipoproteins low-density lipoproteins ratio	nary artery disease

BLOOD CHEMISTRIES:

Increased SGOT, LDH, direct bilirubin	Reason unclear; LDH primarily hepatic and muscle origin
Increased CPK	Primarily muscle origin and may remain elevated for months of high mileage training; apparently not detrimental

ELECTROCARDIOGRAM:

Bradycardia	Training effect, increased vagal tone, increased stroke volume
Primary & secondary AV block, incomplete right bundle branch block (Crista pattern)	Partial heart blocks common among distance runners; apparently not detrimental
Large precordial R-wave, left ventricular hypertrophy by voltage criteria, orthostatic T-wave inversion, early S-T repolarization	Left ventricular mass increased, training effect

STRESS TEST:

S-T depression during exercise	Common abnormality among elite runners; apparently not pathologic

ECHOCARDIOGRAM:

Increased aortic root diameter, increased left ventricular mass, right atrial hypertrophy, increased left ventricular end diastolic volume	Training effects, not apparently pathologic

Common Deviation from Normal	**Comment**
ABNORMALITIES FOUND AFTER LONG DISTANCE RACE SUCH AS MARATHON:	
Increased hematocrit, sodium, chloride, calcium, potassium, BUN, protein, creatinine, uric acid, phosphorus, bilirubin, alkaline phosphatase, CPK, hemoglobinuria and myoglobinuria	Largely reflect dehydration; usually disappear within 1–2 days following hydration.

Suggested Reading

There are very few published studies of runners' medical problems. Therefore, much of the information contained in *The Runner's Medical Guide* is based on our personal experiences. We recommend the following references for those interested in further reading:

Physiology and Training
Astrand, P. O. "Qualification of Exercise Capability and Evaluation of Physical Capacity in Men." *Prog. Cardiovascular Disease.* 19(1), July/August, 1976.
Astrand, P. O., and K. Rodahl. *Textbook of Work Physiology.* New York: McGraw-Hill, 1970.
Dayton, O. W. *Athletic Training and Conditioning.* New York: Ronald Press, 1965.
Howard, H. and J. R. Poortmans. *Metabolic Adaptations to Prolonged Physical Exercise.* Basel: Birkhauer Verlag, 1975.
Jokl, E., and P. Jokl. *The Physiological Basis of Athletic Records.* Springfield: Charles Thomas, 1968.
Jokl, E., and P. Jokl. "Exercise and Altitude." *Medicine & Sport.* S. Karger, ed. Vol. 1, 1968.
Jokl, E. *Physiology of Exercise.* Springfield: Charles Thomas, 1971.
Jokl, E., et. al. "Advances in Exercise Physiology." *Medicine & Sport.* Jokl, S. Karger, eds. Vol. 9, 1976.
Keul, J., et. al. "Energy Metabolism of Human Muscle." *Medicine & Sport.* Jokl, S. Karger, eds. Vol. 7, 1972.

Poortman, J. R. "Biochemistry of Exercise." *Medicine & Sport.* Jokl, S. Karger, eds. Vol. 3, 1969.

Injuries of Runners

Bowerman, J. W. *Radiology and Injury in Sport.* New York: Appleton-Century-Crofts, 1977.

Giannestras, N. J. *Foot Disorders Medical and Surgical Management.* Philadelphia: Lea and Febiger, 1973.

Inman, V. T., ed. *DuVries' Surgery of the Foot.* St. Louis: The C. V. Mosby Co., 1973.

O'Donahue, D. H. *Treatment of Injuries to Athletes.* Philadelphia: W. B. Saunders, 1976.

Pugh, L. G. C. E., *et al.* 1967. "Rectal Temperature, Weight Losses and Sweat Rates in Marathon Running." *Journal of Applied Physiology* 23:347.

Anatomy

Gardner, W. D., and W. A. Osburn. *Structure of the Human Body.* Philadelphia: W. B. Saunders, 1973.

Goss, C. M. *Gray's Anatomy.* Philadelphia: Lea and Febiger, 1959.

Medical Problems

Skin

Demis, D. J., *et al,* eds. *Clinical Dermatology.* Hagerstown, Md.: Harper and Row, 1972.

Ruch, D. M. 1964. "Dermatologic Disorders of Athletes." *Wisconsin Medical Journal* 63:367.

Infections

Hoeprich, P. D. *Infectious Diseases.* Hagerstown, Md.: Harper and Row, 1977.

Tilles, J. G., *et al.* 1964. "Effects of Exercise on Coxsackie Ag Myocarditis in Adult Mice." *Proceedings of the Society for Experimental Biology and Medicine* 117:777.

Respiratory

Bierman, C. W., ed. 1975. "Exercise and Asthma." *Pediatrics* 56:843.

Fitch, K. D., and S. Godfrey. 1976. "Asthma and Athletic Performance." *Journal of the American Medical Association* 236:152.

Morse, J. L. C., *et al.* 1976. "Effects of Terbutaline in Exercise Induced Asthma." *American Review of Respiratory Diseases* 113(1):89.

Paez, P. N., *et al.* 1967. "The Physiological Basis of Training Patients with Emphysema." *American Review of Respiratory Diseases* 95:944.

Scoggin, C. H., *et al.* 1978. "Familial Aspects of Decreased Hypoxic Drive and Endurance in Athletes." *Journal of Applied Physiology* 44:464.

Cardiovascular

Bassler, T., ed. *American Medical Jogger's Association Newsletter* North Hollywood, California.

Cooper, K. H. *The New Aerobics*. New York: Bantam Books, 1970.

Jokl, E. "Heart and Sport." *Medicine & Sport*. Jokl, S. Karger, eds. Vol. 10, 1977.

Kavanagh, T. *Heart Attack (Counter Attack!)*. New York: Van Nostrand Reinhold, 1976.

Milvy, P., ed. 1977. "The Marathon: Physiologic, Medical, Epidemiologic and Psychological Studies." *Annals of the New York Academy of Science* 301:1.

Parker, B. M., et al. 1978. "The Noninvasive Cardiac Evaluation of Long-Distance Runners." *Chest* 73:376.

Sonnenblick, E. H., ed. "Exercise I." *Prog. Cardiovascular Disease*. 18(6), May/June, 1976.

Sonnenblick, E. H., ed. "Exercise II." *Prog. Cardiovascular Disease*. 19(1), July/August, 1976.

Sonnenblick, E. H., ed. "Exercise III." *Prog. Cardiovascular Disease*. 19(2), September/October, 1976.

Gastrointestinal

Bogoch, A. *Gastroenterology*. New York: McGraw-Hill, 1973.

Coyle, E. F., et al. 1976. "Gastric Emptying Rates for Selected Athletic Drinks." *Research Quarterly* 49:119.

Fordtran, J. S., and B. Saltin. 1967. "Gastric Emptying and Intestinal Absorption During Prolonged Severe Exercise." *Journal of Applied Physiology*. 23:1.

Sabiston, D. C. *Textbook of Surgery*. Philadelphia: W. B. Saunders Co., 1972.

Kidneys and Reproductive System

Demos, M. A., et al. 1974. "Acute Exertional Rhabdomyolysis." *Archives of Internal Medicine* 133:233.

Fletcher, D. J. 1977. "Athletic Pseudonephritis." *Lancet* 1:910.

Smith, R. F. 1968. "Exertional Rhabdomyolysis in Naval Officer Candidates." *Archives of Internal Medicine* 121:313.

Ullyot, J. *Women's Running*. Mountain View, California: World Publications, 1976.

Hot Weather

Clowes, G. H., and T. F. O'Donnell. 1974. "Current Concepts of Heatstroke." *New England Journal of Medicine* 291:564.

Knochel, J. P. 1974. "Environmental Heat Illness." *Archives of Internal Medicine* 133:841.

O'Donnell, T. F., Jr. 1975. "Acute Heatstroke." *Journal of the American Medical Association* 234:824.

Pugh, L. G. C. E., et al. 1967. "Rectal Temperature, Weight Losses and Sweat Rates in Marathon Running." *Journal of Applied Physiology* 23:347.

Diabetes

Thorn, G. W., et al, eds. *Harrison's Principles of Internal Medicine*. New York: McGraw-Hill, 1977.

Bondy, P. K. *Diseases of Metabolism.* Philadelphia: W. B. Saunders Co., 1969.

Laboratory Tests

Noakes, T. D., *et al.* 1976. "Biochemical Parameters in Athletes Before and After Having Run 160 Kilometers." *South African Medical Journal* 50:1562.

Riley, W. J., *et al.* 1975. "The Effects of Long Distance Running on Some Biochemical Variables." *Clin. Chim. Acta* 65(1):83.

Miscellaneous

Appenzeller, O. *Pathogenesis and Treatment of Headache.* New York: Spectrum, 1976.

D'Allessio, D. J. 1974. "Effort Headache." *Headache* 14:57.

deWijn, J. F., *et al.* 1971. "Hemoglobin, Packed Cell Volume, Serum Iron and Iron Binding Capacity of Select Athletes During Training." *Journal of Sports Medicine and Physical Fitness* 11:47.

Miller, R. G. 1977. "Transient Focal Cerebral Ischemia after Extreme Exercise." *Headache* 17:196.

Polednak, A. P. 1976. "College Athletes, Body Size and Cancer Mortality." *Cancer* 38:382.

Puranen, J., *et al.* 1975. "Running and Primary Hip Osteoarthritis." *British Medical Journal* 2:424.

Schmid, L. 1975. "Malignant Tumors as Causes of Death Among Former Athletes." *Journal of Sports Medicine and Physical Fitness* 15:117.

Thorn, G. W., *et al.*, eds. *Harrison's Principles of Internal Medicine.* New York: McGraw-Hill, 1977.

Williams, W. J., *et al. Hematology.* New York: McGraw-Hill, 1972.

General Reading

Henderson, J., ed. *Runners' World.* Mountain View, California: World Publications.

Runners' World, eds. *The Complete Runner.* Mountain View, California: World Publications, 1974.

Ryan, A. J., and F. L. Allman. *Sports Medicine.* New York: Academic Press, 1974.

Index

About the Authors

Richard Mangi, M.D., is Clinical Assistant Professor in the Department of Medicine at Yale University School of Medicine, and an established medical investigator with more than fifty scientific publications. He is board certified in internal medicine, infectious diseases, rheumatology and allergy, and immunology. He specializes in medical diseases of muscles and joints and in medical problems of athletes. His interests include infections in athletes and hot weather diseases. Dr. Mangi is an ex-tournament tennis player who now competes as a long distance runner. He is a member of the Sleeping Giant Pacers AAU Running Club with an age group ranking in the state of Connecticut. He has completed more than ten marathons, including the 1978 Boston Marathon in 2:48.

Peter Jokl, M.D., is Director of Athletic Medicine and Assistant Professor of Surgery at Yale University School of Medicine. He is board certified in orthopedic surgery. Dr. Jokl has a lifelong interest in sports medicine and has written numerous articles and books, including *The Physiologic Basis of Athletic Records* and *Exercise and Altitude*. He performs all of the athletic surgery for Yale University. His basic research interests include muscle physiology and injury prevention. Dr. Jokl started competitive running at the age of twelve as a quarter-miler, and competed successfully on championship teams in high school and at Yale University where he held the Ivy League Mile Relay record. He has continued to run regularly and is now a long distance runner, having completed several marathons. He is an active member of the American Medical Joggers Association and a frequent participant in the Honolulu Sports Medicine Conference.

O. William Dayton is athletic Head Trainer Emeritus at Yale University. He is generally considered the dean of American athletic trainers with more than forty years of experience in this field. His career includes: trainer, U.S. Olympic Team, Tokyo 1964; head trainer, University of Miami, Tulane University and Texas A&M; President, Eastern Athletic Trainers Association. He has written two books, *Athletic Training and Conditioning* and *Handbook of Athletic Training*. He is a pioneer in many aspects of the treatment of acute athletic injuries, including taping and rehabilitation.